MW01274405

Wilfried Ehrmann

Coherent Breathing

Aligning Breath and Heart

How to Improve Our
Heart Rate Variability
With Our Breathing

© tao.de in J. Kamphausen Mediengruppe GmbH, Bielefeld
First edition 2017
Author: Wilfried Ehrmann
Cover design, illustration: @graphlight, fotolia
Translation: Wilfried Ehrmann
Proofreading: Annouchka Bayley
Publisher: tao.de in J. Kamphausen Mediengruppe GmbH, Bielefeld,
www.tao.de, eMail: info@tao.de
ISBN:
978-3-96051-538-8 (Paperback)
978-3-96051-539-5 (Hardcover)
978-3-96051-540-1 (e-Book)
First published in German 2016 by Tao-Verlag, Bielefeld,
titled: "Kohärentes Atmen. Atmung und Herz im Gleichklang".

Figures:
Fig. 1-4: ©Wilfried Ehrmann
Fig. 5: Wilfried Ehrmann using ©Bill2499, dreamstime
Fig. 6: ©Wilfried Ehrmann
Fig. 7-8: ©Steven Elliott, with kind permission
Fig. 9-12: ©Wilfried Ehrmann

Wilfried synthesizes complex research from many schools of breathwork in understandable and compelling ways that translate directly to practices critical to controlling our own well-being. He is thorough in his research and documentation while being conversational and accessible in his presentation. In short, he delivers relevant life enhancing information on how we can use our breath to directly change our physical, emotional and mental states for the better. Coherent Breathing puts together theory and scientific data into an easily digestible format for immediate use in our daily lives.

Jim Morningstar, PhD, founder of the School of Integrative Psychology in 1980 and the Transformations Breathworker Training, pioneer in the integration of psychotherapy with such mind/body techniques as breathwork and bio-spiritual energetics, author of four books.

Table of Contents

Foreword

This book deals with the subject of breathing "coherently", a system of breathing that is celebrating its 13th birthday as of this year, 2017. Fundamentally, Coherent Breathing leads the breather to inhale and exhale in a synchronous manner at their *resonant* rate, in combination with conscious relaxation, so as to facilitate wave action in the body. Resonant *coherent* wave action depends on both breathing and relaxation.

If we're familiar with resonance as it relates to the human body, we may be used to thinking of it as "cardio-pulmonary resonance", this because for the last few decades we have been able to observe resonance in the action of the heartbeat easily and non-invasively via plethysmography, where plotting the heart rate in time yields the heart rate variability (HRV) cycle. With the advent of Coherence instruments (2009), we are able to see blood action associated with both breathing and heartbeat, the former being impetus for variability of the latter, the state of the art definition of resonance being the near 180 degree phase correlation of the two phenomena.

A more complete understanding of how one elicits this resonant physical state reminds us that the central nervous system is also intimately involved, both autonomic and somatic functions thereof. So a more complete way to think of resonance is as a state wherein the body and mind are united in purpose, this purpose being realization and maintenance of a *state of mind/body coherence*. Perhaps Mae-Wan Ho's definition of coherence is most complete, this being that coherence is an expression of wholeness of a living system, where it's opposite, incoherence, is a measure of its entropy. Life requires organization and integration; disease and death accrue from its opposite, disorganization and disintegration.

Our present state of understanding is that "healthful" breathing promotes wholistic health and well-being and that poor breathing promotes its opposite. A primary mechanism by which breathing affects our health is by facilitating healthful circulation and its outcome, autonomic nervous system balance, where this balance can be observed via multiple biometrics including EEG, EMG, heart rate, blood pressure, skin conductivity, and hand temperature, where we tend to see these measures shift rapidly toward balance and away from sympathetic dominance once Coherent Breathing begins, autonomic balance swinging like a pendulum from sympathetic to parasympathetic emphasis with each cycle of inhalation and exhalation, respectively. Whether autonomic balance is an outcome of the wave or the wave is an outcome of autonomic balance is a question. What we do know is that the wave is an outcome of synchronous coherent diaphragm movement combined with conscious relaxation.

The current theory is that Coherent Breathing influences central nervous system function by bathing the body and brain with wave-like circulation, this "Valsalva Wave" issuing from the chest during exhalation via the left heart and arterial tree, and returning to the chest via the venous tree and right heart during inhalation. This wave action can be observed almost anywhere a plethysmograph can be attached including arteries, veins, and capillary circulation. The presence of the wave can also be observed in the brain non-invasively via EEG and HEG.

Breathing induced heart rate variability, wherein the heart rate rises coincident with inhalation and falls coincident with exhalation, is an autonomic response to the presence of the respiratory wave via baroreception. I make this distinction because myriad autonomic factors affect heart rate. However, when breathing is synchronous and coherent, breathing tends to dominate and the HRV cycle phase locks with breathing.

The volume and power of heart contractions are also synchronized with breathing so as to accommodate alternating circulatory emphasis, i.e. blood volume rising in the arterial tree during exhalation and rising in the venous tree during inhalation, their overall equality being of critical concern to the autonomic nervous system.

Coherent Breathing, the system, offers a method for breathing and a method for relaxing, so as to elicit *mind/body resonance*, the method of relaxation being "The Six Bridges". The six bridges are anatomical zones that possess both conscious and unconscious governance. They also all exhibit an "open" and "closed" state. The bridges are associated with the parts of the body with which we interact with the world around us, transmitting or receiving, affecting or sensing, input or output. Two clearest examples are the eyes and the diaphragm. We have clear conscious control of each, but when we are not controlling them consciously, the autonomic nervous system controls them for us – automatically.

So Coherent Breathing, the system, proposes that we *learn* or re-learn to breathe and to relax *consciously* so as to generate the wave in the mind/body. Having trained both properly, it becomes automatic – not unlike riding a bicycle. It becomes a choice that we may make mindfully.

My many thanks to Dr Wilfried Ehrmann for bringing the theory and practice of Coherent Breathing to German speaking people around the world.

Stephen Elliott, Life Scientist, Author

Author's Note

For a long time, I have been intrigued by conscious breathing. For the first time in my life, I explored the power of breath by learning to play the clarinet at the age of 11. Suddenly, my breath could produce sounds with the help of the instrument, and the quality of these sounds depended on the length and strength of the breath, whether they sounded strong and clear or weak and dwarfed. Also the beauty of the tone was the result of the flow of breath.

Many years later I started to develop an interest in my inner world. I took therapy for years and visited groups for self-development. I felt drawn to body therapy when I realized that therapeutic talking alone could not bring me deep enough into myself. During this time, I had my first experience with conscious connected breathing in a longer session, which connected me to deeper layers of my psyche. Since then the passion for breath consciousness has not left me. I started to work as psychotherapist and connected the awareness and mindfulness of breathing with other approaches I had been trained in. I noticed the important role of breathing in bringing up and resolving inner issues with myself and with many clients throughout close to thirty years of practice.

Together with colleagues I founded an association in Vienna dedicated to fostering and spreading breathwork in different forms. Since the early nineties, it has grown to a considerable organization with various activities. I am the editor in chief of a journal on breath therapy and breathwork and have been facilitating a training program for breathworkers since 1993. In 1995, I came into contact with the international scene of conscious breathing and have been working for the *International Breathwork Foundation* since then.

After having written several dozens of articles about the breath and about breathing, I started to write a basic manual of breathwork, which was published as "*Handbuch der Atemtherapie*" in 2005 (parts of the book have been translated into English and can be obtained from the author). Since then, a decade has passed, and new developments arose in the world of the breath, with new insights and methods.

In 2011, I completed my second book, which is also available in English: "Consciousness in Evolution". It describes the history of mankind and its traces in the souls of humans from an integral perspective. By this I came into contact with integral forums, where people are occupied with evaluating, interpreting and improving the vast work of the US philosopher Ken Wilber. There I met Günter Enzi, who one day talked about Coherent Breathing, in which he was interested in its connection to heart rate variability.

With his selfless support I started to explore intensely the relationships between the rhythm of the heartbeat and breathing. Soon I noticed in my own investigations how easily and quickly Coherent Breathing could calm me down and help me to relax profoundly. I could prove the physiological efficiency of the method by measuring the improvements in the figures of my heart rate variability.

Out of the cooperation with Günter, the idea to this book was born. He supported me with a lot of precious hints during the process of writing. I am very grateful for his contribution to the book. I contacted Stephen Elliott, the founder of Coherent Breathing, who welcomed my project spontaneously and gave me a lot of professional help with several questions, which came up in the process of writing. I also thank him warmly for the preface to this book.

My own experiences and those of many clients and students have strengthened my conviction that Coherent Breathing can be an invaluable help for relieving and healing many if not all the problems and sufferings of our bodies and souls. This is why I hope that this book will help many people who are interested in the breath on their way and that it will inspire many to become interested in the breath. Being interested in one's breathing always implies being interested in one self, one's body and spirit, health and inner balance.

On Reading this Book

The method of Coherent Breathing, which is presented and explained in this book, is easy to understand and to practice. You might ask yourself why so much theory is necessary and opt instead to turn directly to the relevant chapter on the method itself and begin practice.

There is nothing wrong with this as not all need to be pleased and enthusiastic about theoretical insights. I tried to keep the excursions to physics, biology and chemistry as simple and easy to grasp as possible. There is a glossary of special terms at the end of the book. And those who want to get more information about certain aspects of the manifold connections, which are important for Coherent Breathing, can use the references for deepening the knowledge about the subject.

For understanding, why Coherent Breathing should be practiced in one way and not in another, as described in this book, it is crucial to comprehend the background. Otherwise, someone might have the idea to make the exercises "intuitively" in a different way, which is not fundamentally wrong but misses the deeper effects of Coherent Breathing.

Apart from that, understanding what is going on in the body when breathing is aligned to a coherent rhythm can enhance the inner effects because we have an intimate connection between cognition and organic processes. We need an insight about the usefulness of new exercises; otherwise the motivation can fade away soon.

Many people have a visual access to the inside of their bodies. Knowing about the internal processes and connections can help to connect the breathing exercises with imagination and visualization, which can help to easier dive into the desired rhythm.

Finally, it helps spreading the method when we gain an understanding about its impact on our physiology and our well-being. Many people in our culture need a theoretical background as assurance to enter into new ways of perception and experience or unfamiliar practices. Far too quick, we tend to remove methods, which do not stand up to the rigid demands of science, to the corner of speculation or esoterics. Yet, this book gives nourishment for both: Those who want to give a try to a new method, and those who first have to soothe their inner critic before going into practice.

In the initial chapter, I describe a new paradigm, which is probably necessary for the whole area of health services and will become more urgent in near future as it is about viewing ourselves not only as consumers of public health care, but as primary responsible for our own health. The method presented in this book claims to offer an important contribution to this new orientation, which everyone can utilize as long as one is able to breathe consciously. But it needs a widely socially accepted basis in form of a scientifically verified and at the same time sufficiently comprehensible theory.

The general remarks of the first chapter are presented in more detail in the second. The model of the polyvagal theory helps to understand the central role of our autonomic nervous system for our well-being and our social competence and how we can influence it beneficially.

The third chapter offers an explanation of coherence, a pheno-menon already existing in inanimate objects striving for interactive harmony. Even more, we can take advantage of the notion of coherence in regard to processes in our bodies, because health and coherence seem closely interlinked. In this context, we will deal with heart rate variability, which offers a yardstick for this connection.

The fourth chapter leads us to the connection of heartbeat and breathing rhythm and thus to the immediate preparation for Coherent Breathing. Here we find the new discovery by Stephen Elliott and his team: We can shape our breathing in a way that it optimally supports and unburdens the activity of heart and blood circulation. By this, a wave of coherence is activated, which in turn harmonizes many other physiological systems.

Equipped with these provisions, we get to know Coherent Breathing in its practical form to encounter and understand its fundaments in the fifth chapter. Now there is nothing to prevent starting to practice right away, and the next section offers extensive practical hints, recommendations and support. In the seventh chapter, we find further Coherent Breathing exercises, among them the "six bridges", which is an enlargement of Coherent Breathing.

The seventh chapter gives an overview over many breathing methods and schools, which have developed over time, so that we can see the value of Coherent Breathing in a broader context, and we can judge, which breathing exercises are useful for which purposes. Many people use breathing exercises and are familiar with certain methods. It is important for them to understand how their exercises relate to Coherent Breathing.

The eighth section will go into more detail about the chemistry of breathing. It is of great importance for this subject how the physical compression ratios we use in Coherent Breathing are related to the chemical process of the oxygen and carbon dioxide metabolism during breathing.

In the ninth chapter, the connection between breathing and hormone regulation in the body will be explored in respect of the question whether and how rapid and deep breathing can be beneficial for our health.

The tenth chapter presents integrative breathing as comprehensive method of breath therapy and prepares the ground for the next section dealing with the question how especially Coherent Breathing can be used in psychotherapy. Finally, the application of Coherent Breathing in coaching, sports and with children will be highlighted.

The terms "Coherent Breathing" and "Valsalva wave" used in this book are protected by copyright by COHERENCE LLC.

In this book, all male attributions include females and vice versa. Quotations from German sources are translated by the author.

Chapter 1 – Taking Care of Our Health

We are on the edge of a basic shift of our health care system. Many prognoses indicate that we are about to hit the borders of financial viability. The undeniable successes of medical research and practice have brought a lot of alleviation to sick people and prolonged their lives. On the other side, we notice a growing number of illnesses and new forms of diseases, which cause us worries. There is also an increasing dissatisfaction with medical care by many, even in countries with enormous expenses for the health care system. Academic medicine based on classical science can help a lot of people but by far not all. It best works with "normal patients" with average sensitivities and resilience. Others react allergically to medication or cannot tolerate the standard doses. Many suffer from disorders without diagnosis. They run from examination to examination without result. They have "pains without findings". Others suffer from the side effects of treatments more than from the original symptoms.

Medical treatments have to become more individualized: Every patient needs a therapy adjusted to his condition and needs. At the same time, the cost pressure rises and the time doctors can dedicated to their patients decreases. The waiting times become longer, the dissatisfaction grows. Although more and more money is pumped into the system, it seems as if people are not becoming healthier and happier.

The basic shift we are probably facing presently means taking on self-responsibility. We are used to other people caring for our health: doctors, hospitals and the whole social and health care system. Now it is the point to reclaim this responsibility to ourselves without having to renounce the support of experts. We should become the primary experts for ourselves and see the specialists of the health care system as partners.

Medicine of the third person perspective (diagnosing and treating symptoms from outside) needs to be complemented by the first person perspective (investigating symptoms from the inside). So the challenge is to build up and improve our own health competence, and we notice the presentation of more and more promising approaches.

We discover ways to influence our bodies from the inside. For our organism is a gigantic self-controlling system. We know and experience thousands of subsystems regulating themselves all the time. As long as everything runs fine, we do not pay any attention to our blood pressure, lymph circulation or secretion of digestive enzymes. In every moment, our bodies autonomously achieve incredible results. Our brain is taking part in all these procedures. When we want to become the primary doctors inside of ourselves, we should learn to use those parts of our brain as highest authority of inner self-regulation, which are accessible for our consciousness. How can we program ourselves in a way that our bodies remain efficient on the one hand and regenerative on the other?

The method of Coherent Breathing presented in this book offers an important approach to this topic. For with the breathing process, nature has provided us with a metabolic function, which can operate with or without consciousness. With consciousness we can influence the breathing to modulate other physical systems by stimulating or moderating them. We just have to know how to breathe "correctly" for creating the desired results and how we can train our bodies to automatically breathe in a way that is most beneficial for them, which means for us and for our health.

1. The Salutogenetic Concept of Health

We often hear about the crisis of health care. For handling these problems, we presumably need a new paradigm, which includes viewpoints from Salutogenesis. This means:

> „Man is on the way, which is to see as a continuum from health to sickness in many different dimensions and turns away from a dichotomous view of health vs. sickness. With this, we focus on the question, which factors, which coping resources help to manage life, and turn away from a view about stressors, which is loaded with negativity, as stressors can be seen as helpful signals in the life of a person as well. When dealing with stressors, it matters to explore their character and to find ways for the individual to handle them and succeed in resolving the tension." (Lorenz, S. 26)

Crucial is the question, how an organism manages to grow and develop in a healthy way – that is to create a dynamic order, which is named coherence by the founder of Salutogenesis, Aaron Antonovsky. Life involves various challenges the human organism has to cope with. For this task, it needs the ability to regain balance, when imbalance happens due to the influence of different stressors. Thus, it will also improve its general coping abilities.

2. Tow Pillars of Health

Based on these reflections, I would like to present the model of health on two pillars. Human health rests on two mutually dependent perspectives:

- Self-care (first person perspective)
- Professional support (third person perspective)

Self-care and self-competence always should be in the first place: One's own individual awareness of body and health, mindfulness of one's own quality of life, and the ability to handle impairments to this quality, so that the right equilibrium can be restored quickly.

In case of need, when self-competence does not suffice, the public organizations of care with their experts: therapists, doctors, hospitals, pharmacies etc. come into play.

When we take both pillars seriously and appreciate them in their importance, one's own health does not get delivered completely to the health care system as it is the case to a large extent today, which causes high expenditure and human burdens. Rather, the primary and ultimate responsibility stays with the persons concerned, and this should also be acknowledged by the professional health management and by the governmental health policy. This primary and ultimate responsibility can be adopted by the individuals by strengthening their own competence concerning their bodies and their health.

This implies:

- Collecting and using information, i.e. health education,
- Improving one's own life style in areas in which one's well-being is reduced or impaired,

- Setup and cultivation of exercises and practices serving the maintenance of health,
- and continuous attention on the inner perspective, i.e. inner health monitoring.

3. Coherent Breathing as Method for Self-Provision

Coherent Breathing is an easy to learn and universally applicable method for prevention and self-therapy. On the one hand, it helps to balance the nervous system and on the other to strengthen self-awareness and self-perception. It supports us in situations of acute stress to calm down and takes the pressure out of daily experiences. It is useful for our own sense of health: To perceive how we feel with ourselves, to notice when we get out of balance, and to discern what helps us in tense situations and what is detrimental to us.

Every day, hour, minute we are together with ourselves. In any moment of our lives we know how we feel, we just have to ask our inside. What we need is a sense of when we are in inner balance and when we skip out of it. And when we are in imbalance, this the way, which brings us back to harmony and equilibrium. The simplest indicator for inner disturbances and the simplest corrector at the same time, is our own breathing. Breath awareness, that is attention to our own breathing, is a helpful access to our inner world, which is always at hand. The self-regulation by breathing is an excellent way to restore our inner alignment again and again.

It is imperative that we all become the most important experts for our own health! We just have to get started!

So this is the urgent and necessary shift of paradigms in our attitude towards health and quality of life: We can take on more responsibility for our health. Now there are numerous developments within the medical research, which back us up in this task. I mention two interrelated tendencies in this context: The new validation of the vegetative nervous system as basic component in any disease in general and findings about the role of the parasympathicus in stress regulation in particular.

4. The Autonomic (Vegetative) Nervous System

The basic role of the autonomic nervous system in all processes of our bodies and thus in all disorders, which arise, becomes more and more evident. In many cases, it is no more sufficient to just treat the single symptoms of a disease without looking at the general state of the organism. Thus the perspective shifts from single symptoms to the dynamics in the background, which have led up to the rise, maintenance and deterioration of the symptoms.

The particular role of the autonomic nervous system stems from the fact that it is part of the regulation of all physical processes together with the brain. It provides resources and information required for strenuous tasks and steers the systems back to balance afterwards. Yet in case this central system of regulation is over-worked, mismanagement is the inevitable result, leading to various symptoms.

So it makes sense to take the correct functioning of the nervous system into account when treating the different disorders of or-ganismic processes. Despite a momentary relief, symptoms will come back in the same or a different form when the basic physical pro-cesses could not be healed. Yet when the "operating system" is tuned to its optimal performance, it is likely that symptoms do not have to appear any longer and the normal state, which is health, prevails sustainably.

Sympathicus and Parasympathicus

As we know, the autonomic nervous system consists of two main agents, which cooperate mutually, compete sometimes and help each other out at times.

The interplay of the sympathetic and the parasympathetic branch of the nervous system is traditionally simply seen in this way: When the sympathicus is active, the parasympathicus is passive, and the other way round. As the sympathicus is the stress engine of the body, which tunes it up, many endeavors in stress prevention were aimed at the sole goal to calm it down: We just have to manage to come out of the stress mode, and this is all that has to be done for caring for our health. For when the sympathicus is calm, the parasympathicus automatically goes into action and helps us with regeneration.

Yet more and more we learn that sympathicus and para-sympathicus are different systems, which can complement each other well and orchestrate certain processes together like e.g. in breathing or in sexuality. Additionally, both are also individualists with a respective "personality". They can activate and deactivate themselves independently of the other. And they react differently to influences from outside and have their own history. E.g. the parasympathetic system can be weakened from early on, for instance by a difficult birth (Wittling & Wittling 2012, 99f), apart from distortions in pre-natal developmental events during the formation of the nervous system in the course of pregnancy.

Consequently, it is not enough to reduce the stress reaction by throttling the sympathicus. The parasympathicus has to play its role as well, but it does not act automatically by starting its job as soon as the sympathicus is done. Its ability to supply adequate regeneration depends on its own strength.

On the other hand, there is the less frequent case that the parasympathicus is over-activated and the sympathicus is weakened. This constellation was observed with children suffering from attention deficit hyperactivity disorder[1].

From psychotraumatology we know that an over-active state of the parasympathetic system is connected with freezing, extreme help-lessness and dissociation. In the chapters 2 and 11 we will go into more detail about this. In this constellation, the strengthening of the sympathetic system is required to balance the parasympathicus.

So we need both: a strong and flexible sympathicus to be able to act and a strong and flexible parasympathicus to be able to re-generate. Even if we have learned to calm down our stress engine, this is not enough for recreation. Our complete inner balance needs a parasympathicus with sufficient "power".

For constant stress does not only weaken the sympathicus, but also damages the parasympathicus. When stress becomes chronic, the parasympathetic system can only become active in niches like extended holidays. Thus its power fades, and the body becomes less and less able to regenerate. It gets increasingly difficult to come down after a strenuous day.

5. Strengthening Para-Power and Total-Power

How can we figure out the state of our nervous system? The degree of activation of the sympathetic nervous system can be measured relatively easily by measuring the acute stress level via the cortisol level in the blood. Also the blood pressure reflects the degree of sympathetic arousal. Yet for a long time, there was no simple procedure to detect the parasympathetic activity. Only with the pro- gress of non-invasive measurement of heart rate variability since the beginning of the nineteen nineties, could reliable and relatively easy accessible data be collected. Due to this we are able nowadays to improve our understanding of the general peculiarities and reactive patterns of the autonomic nervous systems. Furthermore we can demonstrate with rather simple means to any individual how her nervous system reacts and where its strengths and weaknesses are.

For many of us it will be important to find ways to strengthen the parasympathicus, the para-power to become more stress-resilient, as stressful experiences and emotional strain affect the efficiency of this system, which is so important for our well-being and long lasting stability. Yet, as already mentioned, also the sympathicus can be impaired, so that we always have to look at the whole picture of our autonomic nervous systems, the so-called total-power.

Our next question is dedicated to the possibilities of influencing the autonomic nervous system. How can we balance its deficits and strengthen it in a way that it optimally supports our health and per- formance?

This book presents Coherent Breathing as one of these possi- bilities. There are a lot more: nutrition, motion (endurance sports), time in nature and sufficient sleep, just to name a few. Breathing plays a key role, as it is the only metabolic process, which works uncon- sciously on the one hand and can be observed and altered consciously on the other hand. In addition to that, breathing is closely interconnected with the autonomic nervous system, by which it is modulated and regulated; and reciprocally we can moderate our nervous system by consciously initiating changes of our breathing pattern. So breathing offers us the chance to directly monitor our vegetative state and to navigate it according to our intentions and needs.

6. Practice Creates Health Competence

If we want to implement long lasting changes in the vegetative processes of our bodies, there is just one way: exercise, for we want to change reflexes, habitually established and fixated behavioral patterns, and this only works when we practice the new patterns on and on until our bodies make them part of their spontaneous repertoire. Our organisms are conservative systems, which need endurance and consistency to change their processes.

We always should keep in mind that our organisms had to cope all the years with our habits and carelessness and had to adjust to them. They had to find compromises at times and gradually deviated from the norm of optimal functioning. Yet as long as the reserves were sufficient for carrying on, the relevant activities were rated as successful and turned into habits, as habitual processes are "cheaper", consuming fewer resources by running in the same way all the time. On the other hand, the organism keeps them up stubbornly, even when it starts to work against itself as it is e.g. obvious in auto-immune diseases.

Disorders as Messages

Overloading our nervous capacities creates habitualized compensations. The effects remain unnoticed often for years or even decades, until it gets too much in one part of the body. Now the body signals that it is unable to readjust itself – by pains, weakness, exhaustion, disease etc. These symptoms are messages stating that parts of our organism need help and they appeal to our consciousness: "By this pain I want to inform you that I am no longer able to cope on my own, I need your support."

We can give this aid to it (us) in a specific or in a general way: Specifically by treating or having treated the disorder and generally by taking the message seriously and deciding to improve our basic condition, so that such disorders cannot happen anymore. This basic condition rests on the equilibrium of our vegetative nervous system, namely on its ability to perform actively and to recover passively after that.

As explained, the basic processes are programmed safely by habitual behavior over years. For a long time, our bodies have formed the belief that things cannot work better than they work. This is why it needs longer to adapt to new habits and to adopt them. We can support this process by noticing progress: Something has changed, I have become calmer, I can relax easier, etc. By this, we initiate positive feedback cycles, which motivate us to stick to the new practices.

E.g. when a former smoker notices how good it feels to mount stairs without coughing, it quickens the decisiveness to stay with the new habits. Perceiving success and positive experiences even works on a deeper level by releasing messenger substances, which support the implemented changes in the nervous system.

Thus we understand why we need with consistency and commitment to reach our goals, which grant us health and fitness, represented by a balanced autonomic nervous system.

Important Points:

We can and we should take over the primary responsibility for our health and well-being.

For this task it is crucial to observe and influence the state of our autonomic nervous system.

This task mainly relates to the ability to calm the sympathicus, and this means that we have to strengthen the parasympathicus.

Coherent Breathing is a method for improving the parasympathicus, which can be trained without big effort and can be practiced at any time and any place.

Chapter 2 – The Polyvagal Theory

1. The Autonomous Nervous System

The autonomic nervous system is the part of the nervous system, which is withdrawn from conscious regulation and control to a large extend. So these processes work without our active support and knowing. Among them are the basic processes of metabolism: breathing and digestion, but also the functioning of the other organs like heart or sexual organs. In this book, we will learn about chances to play our conscious role in the procedures of this part of the nervous system.

Health means that the vegetative nervous system is in a good balance – it can provide the energy necessary for performance and strain and it can sufficiently relax and regenerate. By this, the immune systems are in optimal state and can cope well with the challenges the organism receives from outside.

The vegetative nervous system not only orchestrates our physical functions, but also creates the fundament for our moods. Whether we are tired or awake, active or passive, free or oppressed, depends on the interactions in our nervous system. As it is in charge of releasing or retaining hormones and messenger substances, it forms the fundament for our moods and emotions.

Described in the first chapter, the autonomic or vegetative nervous system can be divided into two branches, which work like a swing: The sympathicus is always there for us for performance and strain, for all kinds of stress (di- and eu-stress). The parasympathicus is our helper for relaxation and provides pleasant states of recreation. When one is at work, the other stays in the background.

Regulated by *hypothalamus*, brain stem and *formatio reticularis*, the nerves of the sympathicus originate from the chest and lumbar sections of the central column. The parasympathicus comes from the brain stem (brain nerves III., VII., IX. and X., the latter being the vagus nerve), and, for the lower belly area, from the sacrum.

A high vagal tonus, i.e. a strong parasympathicus, improves a lot of physical functions, among them the level of blood sugar, blood pressure and digestion. The vagus conveys information from the microbiom in the intestines and cares for correcting reactions to processes of inflammation indicated by pathogen micro-organisms[2].

The regulation of both branches of the vegetative nervous system is divided between the two brain hemispheres. The right hemisphere, which among others has the task of dealing with challenging and threatening situations in the outer world, controls many of the sympathetically modulated processes in the body. As opposed to that, the left hemisphere regulates processes, which decrease environmental stress and further growth and regeneration. For this, it controls the parasympathicus (Wittling & Wittling 2012, p. 80 – 82).

2. The Polyvagal Theory

The polyvagal theory broadens the classical view of the autonomic nervous system. It was first presented in 1996 by the US-American scientist Stephen Porges. Since then, a lot of follow-up research was conducted and practically tested in different areas. The theory states that in mammals the vagus has two parts, and both fulfill quite different roles, although both are central for the parasympathetic system. There is a dorsal (rearward) and a ventral (front) branch. Physiologically, there is a difference as the ventral branch is myelinated, i.e. covered by an isolating sheath, so it can react quicker as the unmyelinated dorsal vagus.

The new discovery by Stephen Porges consists in the finding that the ventral, new or also "smart" vagus is responsible for the functioning of the social and communicative system (SSE=*system social engagement)*. In fact, all mammals have to care for their newborn offspring, which are totally helpless and dependent. So they have to understand their specific needs and react to them, until they have learned to take care of themselves. Reptiles, which are not equipped with this system, only have to breed their progeny without needing a lot of empathy and communicative skills.

3. The Developmental History of the Nervous System

In terms of evolution, the autonomic nervous system has developed gradually from reptiles to mammals according to Porges.

First there was the vagal system originating from the dorsal nucleus in the brain stem, typical for reptiles. Then the sympathetic ganglia were formed at the side of the spinal column (neural nodes). They are responsible for the maximal mobilization of resources for all situations of threat, basically for the fight-flight mechanism. Finally, a second part of the vagus was formed in mammals. Both parts originate from the brain stem, but gradually detached from each other. The new vagus originating from the ventral nucleus provides the neural regulation of contact and communicative behavior.

The Hierarchy of the Nervous Systems

Smart Vagus (SSE) ventral vagus, vagal brake (blocks sympathicus) - mammals
Sympathicus spine - ganglia activiation, mobilization, stress, fight/flight
Parasympathicus dorsal vagus immobilization, figning death, dissociation

Fig. 1: The hierarchical model of polyvagal theory

These systems are used conversely: In the normal state of functioning, the new "smart" vagus is in operation. When it cannot cope with a certain challenging situation the sympathicus with its mobilizing strategies gets activated. It prepares for fight or flight. In this phase, the communicative skills are widely restricted.

When finally this reactive pattern fails, the old parasympathicus takes over by shutting down all systems. Mammals react by immobilization, fainting, and feigning death up to purging the bowels. This physiologically oldest and most primitive neuronal circuit is mediated by the unmyelinated (dorsal, vegetative) vagus. It provides the last left resources. When these are completely depleted, the organism dies.

4. The Vagal Brake

The "vagal brake" mediates between smart vagus and sympathicus by keeping breathing and heart frequency low. Thus the functioning of the social communication is guaranteed: we are relaxed and can easily connect with other people.

In the same way, the new vagus can moderate the old one. Heart rate and breathing frequency get decelerated rhythmically (mainly in the phase of exhalation). This allows us e.g. to care for our offspring and their needs. When we engage in social contact by listening and talking, we need calmness and safety. These qualities are mediated unconsciously via feedback from the neural nodes in the brain responsible for communication (III, V, VII, VIII, XI, XII). They influence e.g. the facial muscles, which are crucial for nonverbal signals and are closely interlinked with the ventral vagus nucleus.

The Purpose of the Freezing Reaction

Why has the parasympathetic reaction of freezing and feigning death prevailed in mammals? It makes sense with reptiles (diving reaction of a crocodile, restriction of metabolism of a snake). Yet for mammals, this behavioral pattern is dangerous and bears great risks, as the extreme reduction of breathing and heartbeat (*bradycardia*) causes extreme lack of oxygen for the organism. As opposed to reptiles, mammals have a high need of oxygen, and in the parasympathetic state a life threatening shortage is reached quickly. Phenomena like sudden cardiac arrest or nocturnal child death can be caused by deregulated parasympathetic states.

Porges assumes that this form of reaction of the autonomic nervous system has prevailed as it is of use in a different way in social contexts: Motionlessness connected with total surrender can be found in breastfeeding, in certain phases of partnership and in sexuality, especially when there is a strong bond of trust between the partners. This adapted form of reaction is supported by the release of oxytocin, which is produced in the hypothalamus and transported to the dorsal vagus. This is why oxytocin is called the bonding hormone.

5. Vagus and Breathing

The primary regulation of breathing is done by the vegetative nervous system. Calm breathing is the domain of the vagus, stress breathing of the sympathicus. In extreme situations, the vagus in its unmyelinated form takes control and causes the ultimate reduction of breathing up to the point of breathing arrest.

"Physically, breathing restrains the influence of the myelinated vagus on the heart. When we inhale, the influence of the vagus is weakened and the heart rate increases. When we breathe out, the influence of the vagus becomes stronger and the heart rate sinks. This simple mechanical change during breathing strengthens the calming and generally positive impact of the myelinated vagus on the body." (Porges 2010, p. 264, quotes from the German edition)

The shift in the breath regulation can easily be measured as *respiratory sinus-arrhythmia* (RSA) (see chapter 4.2) in a resting state.

Breathing as Indicator of our Mood

Our breath is an unmistakable indicator for our inner state. As soon as the breathing accelerates, the activity of the heart increases, and the stress reaction is triggered. At the same time, the activity of the social system is reduced. We become more and more huffish and start to get on the nerves of other people. In the extreme case, we are blocked, freeze or faint, and drop out of the social system temporarily. So we should be wary of our breathing becoming hectic without physical strain. This is a signal of losing control over the stressful situation and slipping down the hierarchy of vegetative states (Porges 2010, p. 113).

Observations of the respiratory sinusarrhythmia (see. chapter 5.2., p. 55) and the heart rate variability with infants could prove that a well-functioning vagal brake, which is the elaborated skill to integrate stressful situations safely and calm down easily, gives a reliable prognosis for health as well as for social behavior in the future.

Stress-Regulation by Breathing

Our breathing is not just an excellent access for monitoring our inner state, but also the simplest and most brilliant door for the back-regulation of a derailed nervous system. By relaxing our breath, the heartbeat decreases, and eventually the whole stress reaction vanishes. By training our breathing, we can strengthen the ability of our vagus to slow down as soon as the sympathicus is no longer needed. So we swing back to our normal state of relaxation, when the danger is over or when we have realized that the danger was just imagined. Thus we save resources and energy. As soon as we are back in the area of the "smart" vagus, we actively care for our regeneration and health provision, and we are much more pleasant companions for our fellow people.

Rapid and shallow breathing patterns indicate that the heart rate is constantly in the sympathetic realm, and that the vagal brake is no longer or only insufficiently working. This causes a constant burden for the organism, which on the long run can only result in mal-function. Various forms of disorder like depression, epilepsy, autism, schizophrenia and post-traumatic stress disorder have been linked to a weak vagal brake.

So it seems to be a crucial and central access for health provision to strengthen the vagal tonus, thus empowering the parasympathicus. Porges also hopes that in this way disorders like that do not have to be treated by psychotropic drugs, but by methods of breath and body relaxation (Porges 2010, p. 285).

6. Traumatization and the Polyvagal System

We can find the following connection: Calming down and relaxing the breathing improves the activity of the vagus, measurable via respiratory sinusarrhythmia. By this, the activities of the emotional centers in the brain, especially of the so-called fear organ, the *amygdala*, are reduced. Experiments have proved that a stimulation of the vagus nerve leads to an increased activity of the neuro transmitter *gamma-amino-butter-acid* (GABA). This messenger substance is considered the main inhibitor in the brain used for suppressing over-reactions as they occur as consequence of traumatic experiences. Increasing the GABA activity in the insular and prefrontal cortex disables an over-activation of the amygdala and thus reduces fears and anxiety reactions.

Persons suffering from post-traumatic stress disorder (PTSD) show higher sympathetic and reduced parasympathetic arousal. They are in a chronic state of sympathetic over-arousal (Ogden et al., 2006). Similar to autistic people, they avoid direct eye contact and do not react to the human voice. As their vagal brake is defective (probably caused by developmental traumatization) or blocked by an acute traumatization, these persons can only receive limited social signals from their surroundings and consequently their feeling of not belonging and not being understood increases. As primary aid, the improvement of the competence for self-regulation on the level of the nervous system is recommended (see chapter 11.4).

Coherent Breathing is an excellent method for this goal. So it was frequently applied as instrument in trauma treatment in large groups in areas of crisis and with single clients (Brown & Gerberg 2012).

The right part of the vagus nerve is most active in regulating the heart and the basic emotions at the same time. Primary protective emotions like fear, pain and anger (which are also moderated by the right side of the limbic system) require the autonomic functioning of heart and lungs as they originally always carry the responsibility for survival.

The visceral functions are controlled by the brain stem, as soon as there is danger. In this case, higher cognitive functions would be an obstacle as they would limit the mobilization of all resources necessary for survival. This is why in such situations the cortical control of the brain stem is inhibited, while the autonomic structures of the brain stem get disinhibited. Thus the sympathetic nervous system can augment the performance of energy metabolism.

7. The Sensual Organs and Vagal Regulation

Hearing

For the transference of acoustic waves from the eardrum to the inner ear, the auditory ossicles in the middle ear are of specific importance. Two muscles regulate the stiffness of these ossicles: When they are stiff, the transmission of noise with low frequency to the inner ear is reduced or inhibited. Then sounds with higher frequencies can be perceived easier, which is the spectrum of the human voice.

The ossicles are specific for mammals. They help them to communicate with frequencies reptiles cannot perceive. The stiffening mechanism of the middle ear allows communication with human language even when stronger low frequency environmental noise dominates.

The neural regulation of the ossicles is performed by the trigeminus nerve, which co-operates closely with the vagus nerve. The vagal tonus decides whether low frequency environmental noise is preferred or the human voice. When the smart vagus loses its taming grip on the sympathicus, because the environment becomes more dangerous, the frequencies of the human voice cannot be perceived at all or less clear enough. Thus our opportunities for meaningful communication are limited, and misunderstandings happen easily.

Infants with defect stapedius muscles (which can result from middle ear inflammation) can suffer from retardation in language development and even autism.

Seeing

The muscles, which control the eyes and their movements, are regulated by the brain nerves III, IV and VI influenced by the vagus. The eyes are important instruments for social interaction. Nerve tracts in charge of the eye ring muscles are also engaged in the regulation of the middle ear muscles. The articulation of social signals via eye gaze and hearing the human voice are closely interconnected.

The gaze, looking and being looked at play a central role when humans meet and build up trust. The eyes are also called "doors to the soul". On the other hand, we need the eyes for quick orientation in situations of danger. Due to this the eyes perceive other object in another way when under stress: The visual field is contracted, the focus rigid, and the viewing direction is shifted jerkily.

For producing the opposite effect, slowing down the movements of the eyes is used in classical hypnosis and in some methods of trauma therapy (e.g. EMDR). By rhythmically calming down the eye muscles, a state of relaxation is obtained by activating the vagal brake. Thus the aftereffects of burdening experiences on the vegetative nervous system get weakened.

The Voice

The nonverbal part of talking, the melodicism of language, are an important dimension of communication as they convey the emotional content. "It's not what you say, but how you say it," so the proverb. And also in this area, the vagal neural transmissions play a central role and regulate the activities of these systems according to the relevant mood and emotional state.

> "As a whole, the muscles of face and head work as filter, which restricts social stimuli (e.g. observation of the peculiarities of a face and hearing vocalizations) and are crucial factors of engagement in a certain social environment. Neural control of these muscles determines social experience by changing the mimic expression, by influencing the muscles of larynx and pharynx (especially in humans and other primates) and thus regulating the melodics of verbal expressions and attuning the motoric tonus of face and voice via respiratory activity." (Porges 2010, p. 273f)

Mainly by the diaphragm, which plays an astonishingly manifold role in language articulation, but also by other groups of muscles taking part in breathing, verbal expression gets colored emotionally:

> Besides, the breathing frequency is encoded in the phrasing of vocalizations, which can express meaning – independent of the contents of communication. For instance, urgency can be expressed by short phrases in connection with short exhalation (i.e. fast breathing) and calmness by long phrases in connection with long exhalation (i.e. slow breathing." (Porges 2010, p. 274)

It was proven that slow and relaxed breathing connected with emotionally expressive vocalization could soothe the heartbeat via the myelinated vagus, like when singing lullabies to babies (Porges 2010, p. 222).

8. Summary

According to Stephen Porges we have a predesigned hierarchy for the reactions of the nervous system to challenges: The evolutionary newer systems block the older ones. The newest circular process serves to produce states of relaxation and self-sedation. When this does not work, we use the sympathetic-adrenaline system for mobilizing the fight/flight mode. And ultimately we fall back on the old vagal system for freezing and breaking down.

This state originally designed for reptiles can be dangerous for mammals. When there is an overdose of the freezing reaction, this is a peril to life. However, a high charge of the new vagus system is beneficial for emotional processes like mating behavior, sexual arousal and creation of long-term social relationships. For this, feelings of security and trust have to be developed, and these qualities are provided by the vagus system of mammals with the hormones oxytocin and vasopressin. They are produced in the hypothalamus stimulated by the vagal nuclei in the brain stem.

By using our higher cognitive functions for calming the stress reaction, we are open for a good connection to others with facial expression, eye contact, adjusted voice and open ears. Thus we strengthen the influence of the younger vagus, which relaxes us by switching off the stress reaction and making our metabolism more efficient. The soothing influence on heart and lungs additionally serves our health, and both exert their moderating influence on the stress axis.

9. An Extended Model of the Vegetative Nervous System

As clear and helpful as the hierarchical model of stress states in the vegetative nervous system according to Porges is, there is an important connection vital for a broader understanding of our ways of behaving and reacting missing. We do not only use the sympathicus and the dorsal vagus, which is the "belly parasympathicus" in situations of stress for fight or flight, respectively for freezing, but also in relaxed conditions. Furthermore, for comprehension of health, it is crucial to pay attention to a good balance of activities between sympathically and parasympathically oriented, e.g. by phases of motion and of rest. When we exert ourselves in endurance sports or engage in yoga postures, we expose our bodies to a stress experience not connected with a scenario of threat but with circumstances, which are under our control. This context will be explained in more detail in chapter 12.2, p. 146.

So basically we utilize our autonomic nervous system for two categorially different situations: For states of threat and for states of safety. In life, there will often be situations of transition, phases of decision, which category our nervous system will choose. But there is always a strong tendency as to which perspective will be preferred.

So a slight feeling of unsafety can signal that a possible source of danger is being perceived, which proves then as harmless, like in the well-known example of the rolled up rope that looked like a snake in twilight. The stress reaction sets in quickly and gets calmed down by the vagal brake in a short time. For example, if someone does not find his key after leaving the apartment, nervousness creeps up inside and relaxes as the key appears in the side pocket of the coat. But even in these examples we experience the categorical difference of states: Just now we are cheerful and happy, and all by sudden we lose our equanimity and calmness and are in a state of alarm. Our breathing and our heartbeat accelerate, the body temperature changes (we feel hot or cold), we start to sweat etc.

I suggest a model of five states of the autonomic nervous system divided in two categories: states of growth and states of protection. States of growth are characterized by inner and outer safety. The organism is in a coherent flow with phases of expansion (physical or mental strain and achievement, creativity and problem solving) and phases of regeneration (relaxation and recreation). The system social engagement (SSE) is active, communication and interaction thrive, ideas are born and brought to life. The states of protection are characterized by inner and outer menaces, which require the mobilization of resources for saving survival. The organism comes into a state of stress, which leads to reducing or shutting down the SSE. At first, the sympathicus is dominating; when it does not succeed in mastering the danger, the dorsal, old parasympathicus takes over.

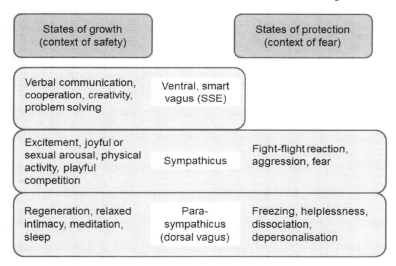

Fig. 2: The Extended Model of Polyvagal Theory

A similar model was proposed by Beth Dennison[3], however, I deviate from this in the following aspect: Dennison assigns a component of threat also to the smart vagus. I refer here to Porges, who allocates the higher social functions to the ventral vagus system, serving community-building among humans. The forces behind posing, greed and workaholism are related to states of protection in my model, as they are driven by fears and rely on a scenario of threat. So they have to be regulated by the sympathicus.

This model corresponds also with the classification of human emotions in feelings of growth and of protection (or expansive and protective feelings according to Müller-Schwefe 2007), which I have explained elsewhere (Ehrmann 2014, p. 24 - 26).

When we understand this model, it becomes clear that we have to take into account both sides of our nervous system, if we want to care for our inner balance. For our health and for the design of our lives we need the expansion of our space for possibilities, that is flexibility in the sympathetic as well as in the parasympathetic area. Flexibility means to fully engage in each of the systems and to withdraw according to the relevant demands of the situation.

Important Points:

Our autonomic nervous system is hierarchically structured: The oldest part is the parasympathicus, followed by the sympathicus, and after that, the new vagus system emerges.

For our communicative and social proceedings we need the new vagus system, which is able to regulate the sympathicus (vagal brake).

When under stress, or dealing with difficult emotional states, the nervous system switches back to older systems so that we enter into the fight/flight mode of the sympathicus and ultimately into the freezing reaction of the parasympathicus.

The stress reaction restricts our sensual perception (hearing and seeing) as well as facial expression, gesticulation and verbal language.

Chapter 3 – What is Coherence?

In this section, a few basic concepts will be explained, which are important for understanding Coherent Breathing: What is coherence in physics and in humans, what is heart coherence and Coherent Breathing and what does heart rate variability mean? The latter will be explained in more detail.

1. What does Coherence Mean?

In physics, the notion of coherence is used to describe the attitude of waves to follow a common fixed pattern in dynamic course. Waves with a stable phase relationship, where up- and downswings are aligned, are called coherent. E.g. the light emitted by a laser is coherent in space and in time.

In the classical physical experiment metronomes are put on a board hanging free to move. The metronomes are tuned in a slightly different rhythm. After a short while of time, all the metronomes are ticking in exact the same rhythm, they have found an agreement, they have created coherence in self-organization.

The experiment points at a phenomenon that nature is able to regulate itself by feedback even in the physical realm and that by doing so, it tends to favor coherent vibrations. From the chaos of different rhythms, an order emerges by itself without any influence from outside. It seems as if the metronomes want to come in harmony with one another. This small experiment demonstrates that there is a strong tendency to harmony and order in nature, even in unanimated elements.

Physics can show that a coherent system is more likely to influence an incoherent one and lead it to coherence rather than the other way around. In doing so, the differing frequencies synchronize and create a coherent vibration. This phenomenon does not only work between objects, but can presumably transposed to sentient beings and especially to humans (Grimm 2015, p. 101). The model of quantum coherence offers additional insights for this idea.

2. Quantum Coherence According to Mae-Wan Ho

The biologist and environmental activist Mae-Wan Ho has developed a comprehensive model of the internal information transfer in organism and especially in humans. It is based on the liquid crystals, which can be found in all cellular membranes (Collings 2001, p. 187-189). These structures are said to be able to spread signals in high speed and in wave form. The network of liquid crystals is evolutionary older than the nervous system and cooperates with it.

For this communication to work efficiently, e.g. in rapid processing of perceptive data and coordination of complexes of movement, a coherent wave form is required. The liquid crystals align to this vibration similar to the pendulums in the physical experiment. As this state is relatively stable, it acts as good attractor, i.e. the system tends to return to the primary state after disturbances by itself. Thus the liquid crystal coherence can serve as fundament of the phenomenon discussed in the next section: The sense of coherence as described by Antonovsky.

According to Mae-Wan Ho, the wholeness of the organism is based on a high degree of quantum coherence. In pure undisturbed form it appears very rarely: "It may be attainable only under very exceptional circumstances, as during an aesthetic or religious experience when the 'pure duration' (...) of the here and now becomes completely delocalized in the realm of no-time and no-space." (Mae-Wan Ho[4]) This is why quantum coherence exists in different degrees or gradation. But we are equipped with the inner urge to strive for the coherent state and to deepen it. Our organism is looking for this coherent state by itself as it is best for its growth and performance.

This is the potent helper in all healing processes: The organism wants to return to its optimal dynamic equilibrium, it wants to increase and enlarge it. All we have to do is to get out of the way and remove all obstacles. Then the coherent state is created by itself, in which we are in harmonious alignment with ourselves and our environment. In meditation and in Coherent Breathing we open the doors for quantum coherence, for the flowing wavelike communication of liquid crystals, according to Mae-Wan Ho's theory.

3. The Sense of Coherence in Salutogenesis

Aaron Antonovsky (1979), founder of Salutogenesis, which has already been mentioned in the first chapter, has described man as a being that is situated on a point on a continuum between health and illness all the time, at one time closer to health and at other closer to sickness. Life consists of mastering challenges. For this, a sufficient amount of resources is required, and among them, the by him so-called sense of coherence has a specific significance.

This sense of coherence is an attitude towards life with three components, which are beliefs:
1. *Comprehensibility*: The world and its events can be understood and reasonably predicted.
2. *Manageability:* The challenges in life are manageable and within control.
3. *Meaningfulness*: Things in life are interesting and a source of satisfaction.

So Antonovsky takes coherence as the alignment of the individual with her surroundings: How far am I in harmony with myself and the conditions and challenges of my life? The more this works, the more likely well-being there is, while any discrepancy causes disorders and diseases. Thus, Antonovsky advocates a holistic view of health by enlarging the view from superficial symptoms to underlying structures. We rather have to focus on general attitudes towards life than on strategies for acute problems and challenges.

Antonovsky states that the sense of coherence exerts a direct influence on different organic systems, e.g. the hormonal and the immune system, as it takes part in deciding whether a certain situation is to be considered dangerous or harmless. It also supports the necessary alterations in case of a distortion and to optimally utilize the available resources (Wydler et al. 2010).

4. Complete Coherence According to Alan Watkins

Alan Watkins, British neuro scientist and management trainer, has presented a comprehensive model of coherence. He claims that we only can preserve our health and produce optimal achievements in our lives when we develop coherence on all levels: In behavior, thinking, feeling, in the emotional area and on the level of physiology. And the latter is the fundament of all. So when the body is not in balance, all the other levels are of no help to keep us in good mood and to act correctly.

For Watkins, coherence is a state of "stable variability" (Watkins 2014, p. 10), consisting of two aspects: the amount and the pattern of variability. This state is the prerequisite of health and creativity. To create this state on the level of the organism, it is crucial to strengthen the coherence of the heart (see next point), for the heart with its oscillations is the strongest pulse generator of the body, which can synchronize all the other rhythms (ibid., p. 43). The heart in turn can be tuned to coherence by breathing:

> "One of the primary ways that we lose our energy is through incoherent or erratic breathing. In the same way that we use more fuel driving in the city than we do driving on the motorway, when our breathing is chaotic we use up much more energy. Coherent Breathing is like motorway driving – we travel further using less fuel, and there is less wear and tear on our system so we feel younger." (ibid., p. 64)

5. Heart Coherence

Not too long ago, the model of coherence got implemented in the organic area (Servan-Schreiber 2004). The idea is that chaotic processes create instability in the body and derange various meta-bolic processes. In contrast, coherently running processes act as positive influence and help us to stay healthy and balanced.

Especially the activity of the heart has been investigated from this point of view. Heart coherence means the even changes of heartbeat intervals. When these changes are regular, i.e. the intervals between the heartbeats become longer and shorter in a regular pattern, the heartbeat is coherent. The alterations show a pattern of regular change. Erratic variations are called chaotic. On a monitor we can see them as a jagged line.

Is there little or no change, when the heart beats as exactly as a metronome, the heart is under extreme stress. This is why an old Chinese saying states: "When heartbeat becomes as regular as the knocking of the woodpecker or the dribbling of rain on the roof, the patient will die within four days." (Wang Shu-he, Chinese physician, 1700 years ago.)

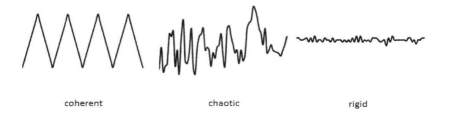

coherent   chaotic   rigid

Fig. 3: Patterns of variability (schematic)

So there is an area of stable or regular variability between chaos and rigid accuracy, a dynamic equilibrium or a constantly self-regulating harmony, which we can call heart coherence.

The coherent heart can adapt to changes much better. It quickly reacts to differing demands from the environment: It speeds up during stress and regenerates during phases of recreation. It registers even small shifts in feelings and moods and balances them. It absorbs the vicissitudes of life and helps us in coping with them, mostly without our noticing by re-establishing a coherent state.

When the heart is in balance, then, as demonstrated by various studies:

1. Blood pressure is lower,
2. Less energy is consumed,
3. Ageing is decelerated,
4. Immune defense is improved,
5. Susceptibility for fears and depression is reduced,
6. Emotional coping with the challenges of life is improved.

An overstrained heart is increasingly less able to manage changes. As a consequence, high blood pressure, diabetes, cancer and cardio-vascular diseases are favored. A deficit in heart coherence and varia-bility can predict a later outbreak of a disease or drastic exacerbation.

In the worst case, it is a very dangerous signal, when the heart no longer reacts to emotional shifts: When heart rate variability has vanished completely, a sudden cardiac arrest and death is highly likely.

As normally seen, sympathicus and parasympathicus are equally responsible for the regulation of the heartbeat, these variation are created by their interplay. In tendency, the sympathicus simplifies the distances between the heartbeats, while the parasympathicus renders them more flexible. To be specific, it can react quicker to changes.

The absence of these variations indicates that the sympathicus alone has taken over control of the heartbeat, and this is risky for the organism in the long run, because it works under high tension and tends to use up all resources. The heart loses its ability to react in an appropriate and well-adjusted manner to the environment and has more troubles in bringing itself back to a regenerative state.

According to studies, coherence immediately affects the performance of the brain and its functions. This results, for example, in quicker reactions and better achievement under stress.

6. Heart Rate Variability

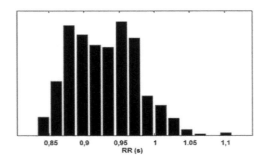

Fig. 4: Frequency distribution of distances between heartbeats in a 10 minutes coherent breathing exercise

Thus we have reached the notion of heart rate variability, abbreviated HRV. The knowledge about this phenomenon spreads rather slowly. The US-American medical scientist Ary Goldberger has stated: the healthy heartbeat "is one of the most complex signals in nature".[5] During a conference in 2002, he showed four different trajectories of heartbeats and asked the audience, which one they would wish for themselves. Most of them, included cardiologists, opted for totally regular curves, which had actually been recorded from patients with severe heart problems.

The term heart rate variability signifies the ability of our heart to react appropriately and flexibly to different demands. The heart reacts in close cooperation with the autonomic nervous system. It slows down the *heart frequency*, and consequently the heart beats at times faster and at times slower. So the *distances between the single heartbeats* vary (in the area of thousandths of seconds), and this is called *heart rate variability*. When the heart beats 70 times/minute (heart frequency=70), we tend to think that the heart beats exactly and regularly. Yet in fact, and that is a good sign, there can be shorter intervals between some beats (e.g. 61.3 heart beats per minute) and longer between others (e.g. 78.7 bpm or 79.7 bpm).

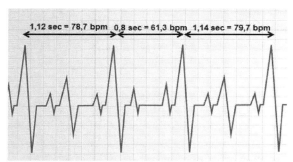

Fig. 5: The variable heartbeat (schematic)

The amount of variability indicates the adaptive potential of the heart and the general state of health. The higher the variability of the heartbeat, the better the nervous system can react to challenges and relax afterwards. As the heartbeat is governed by the autonomic nervous system, the heart rate variability also reports on its condition, especially on the state of the parasympathicus.

In the nineteen-eighties, heart medicine aimed at making the heartbeat as regular and constant as possible. All irregularities should be excluded as they might be dangerous. Meanwhile it has been proven that a healthy heart needs a healthy degree of convertibility and ability to change. *Variatio delectat*, as the Romans said, variety is delicious, and when we are delighted, our heart reacts in diverse ways, while it becomes more stubborn and monotonous in case of anger and tension.

Heart rate variability is age-dependent. It is highest at birth and lowest when we die. In between, there is a constant decline. However this decline in flexibility can be influenced. When we train our lung-to-heart-coherence, the nervous system can rejuvenate. We can commit ourselves to creating a lower coherence age than our actual age. A study from the USA has indicated this potential, where after training for 30 minutes daily over four weeks, the level of the so called youth hormone DHEA was increased by an average of 100 percent[6].

There are other studies, which show that the rhythms of heart and breathing synchronize, when the test subjects focus on feelings like gratefulness and love. On the other hand, the balance between heart and breathing disappears as soon as the subjects think of feelings like anxiety (for example cause by time pressure), anger or fear[7].

Other findings state the effects that even light depression has on reducing heart rate variability, which in turn is an indicator for a higher risk of dying from cardiac disease. Depressions are often linked with heart diseases, and this shows the influence of the breath-heart-system on the general constitution of the whole organism.

7. Measuring Heart Rate Variability

Measuring and interpreting heart rate variability is a science of its own. For it is difficult to convert constant changes into numbers, which should show this convertibility and make it comparable. Heart rate variability is not a simple measure like body temperature, but it is a multidimensional phenomenon, which can be seen and presented from different viewpoints. For this reason, I have presented a variety of different methodologies of measurement in the next section.

Readers who are not interested in these details can skip this section without the danger of missing essential information about the subject of this book.

In many of the thousands of publications on heart rate variability and its various effects on our organism in health and fitness, the figures are presented as if the measurement of HRV would be as simple as measuring the pulse or the blood pressure. But usually, the researches use just one of the various parameters presented here for gaining comparable numbers.

Methods of Measurement

Technically seen, there are the following measuring devices: Pulse measurement, chest strap and ECG.

For measuring heart rate variability exactly, a device monitoring the pulse at the wrist is far too imprecise. Yet there are heart rate monitors, small computer watches, which get their data from a chest strap and work with a resolution of milliseconds sufficient also for scientific purposes. Working with smaller resolution does not result in more accuracy, while a sampling rate under 500 per second creates too much measurement errors.

Measuring with a chest strap and wrist computer is appropriate for hobby practitioners and also affordable. Electrocardiographic measuring is more elaborate and expensive: 12 leads and ten cables are required for a resting ECG and three leads with five cables for a 24 hours ECG. However there are simpler HRV devices working with one lead and one cable for use in 24 hours measurement.

8. Methods of Calculation

Time Domain

Time domain refers to variation of amplitude of signals with time. Initially, the average heartbeat is measured during a certain period of time. Yet this does not describe the degree of variability. So more complex statistical operations are applied to express the deviations from the average.

RMSSD (*root mean square of the successive differences*): Root of the mean of the sum of squares of differences between all successive R-R-intervals. RMSSD informs us about the amount of change of the heart frequency from one heartbeat to the next. This variable is an indicator of parasympathetic activity. It is prone to error with artefacts and rhythm distortions. When below 10 connected with a SDNN value below 20, there is a high risk for cardiac disease.

SDNN: standard deviation of all normal R-R-intervals (total variability). This variable expresses all cyclical components of variability, the "total power" of the regulative system. It also decreases over the course of life: Young people have an average value of 55 and people over sixty of 27.8.

pNN50: counts those gaps between heartbeat peaks, which are more than 50 ms apart. It is an indicator of parasympathetic activity.

Frequency Domain

The high oscillations of the heart frequency can be extracted with a specific operation (*Fourier transformation*) according to certain frequency bands (high, low, very low)[8]. These sinusoidal oscillations contained in the heartbeat can be assigned to certain systems in the body: blood circulation rhythms, blood pressure rhythms, breathing rhythms[9].

Rapid oscillations are produced by the influence of the ventral vagus,, which is able to transmit rapid neural signals, so they are attributed to the parasympathicus. Slower changes come from the sympathicus nerves with their slower conductivity.

Three frequency bands are differentiated, similar to radio waves: The **high frequency band** (HF), the **low frequency band** (LF) and the **very low frequency** (VLF).

The **high frequency band** (*Power HF-Band*) is generally accepted as measure for the activity of the parasympathicus, that is the so-called para-power. It measures the power density spectrum of >0.15 to 0.40 Hz in ms^2. This frequency range corresponds to the respiratory sinusarrhythmia, the rise and fall of the speed of the heartbeat parallel to inbreath and outbreath, cf. chapter 4.2, p. 55.

The **low frequency band** (LF) between 0.04 and 0.15 Hz reflects a mixture of activities performed by sympathicus and parasympathicus. Some time ago, it was considered a reliable measure of the sympathicus, yet in the meantime it became clear that in this band the activities of both branches of the autonomic nervous system are present. This is why the relationship between LF-band and HF-band (HF/LF) is only of minor significance: While the HF-range is a reliable indicator of the parasympathicus, the LF-range contains mixed regulations. The higher the LF-value, the more activities of the sympathicus occurred during the measurement.

The **very low frequency band** (VLF) between 0 and 0.04 Hz is mainly used with 24-hour long measurements and does not play a role in short time measures. Yet it is interesting for measuring the thermo-regulation, which is the control of the regulation of the body temperature[10].

LF/HF-Relation

This variable designates the relation between low and high frequencies and points at the balance of the sympathetic and the parasympathetic system. Higher values either indicate a higher sympathetic or a lower parasympathetic power.

Non-linear Dynamics

In this complex area of HRV measurement, which is reserved for specialists because of its mathematical and statistical peculiarities, the variable D2 is interesting for practical purposes. It reflects the correlation dimension, which measures the system complexity with regard to the degrees of freedom. The more complex a non-linear system behaves, the higher the numeric value of the correlation dimension is. The more variable the heartbeat is, the more complex is the system in mathematical terms. So it is not surprising that patients with cardiac problems have a low D2 value. Scientific research has shown that healthy people have a higher D2 value than patients with high blood pressure and people with heart transplantation who show an even lower value. In healthy people, the value is lower during the day than at night, while this difference cannot be found with hypertonic patients[11]. Another study demonstrated that the variable D2 allows the most exact indication for chronic stress among all HRV variables.

Furthermore, the **Poincaré-Plot** is sometimes used for visualizing the heartbeats and their variability. The successive heartbeats are displayed as point clouds in the plot.

General Remarks:

Generally it is important to note that HRV measurement cannot be universalized due to the complexity of the phenomenon and the relevant factors of influence a single measure during a short period of time (usually five minutes). We know from blood tests that a certain value may be out of the normal range as there is an acute imbalance in a certain metabolic system, which will regulate itself after a short while. Similar to that, a single HRV measurement can be manipulated by different influences – even thoughts about unpleasant events or unresolved problems can lead to higher values in the sympathicus activities.

So it is recommended to repeat HRV measurement under similar conditions (same time, same activities etc.) for gaining relevant data for comparison. After some days of measurement, an average can be stated, and after some weeks of practice e.g. with Coherent Breathing, trends can show the improvement in the various parameters of heart rate variability.

A 24 hour HRV measurement can impressively demonstrate how the values change dynamically in the course of the day, depending on the phases of activity and rest. It provides clear hints as to how far the organism is able to regenerate during the day and especially during the night, that is how the parasympathicus is efficient at night, adding to the immense regenerative value of sleep.

Even though single measures do not allow absolute extrapolations, unusually low values of HRV in different domains, relative to one's age, should be a cause of concern. For a very low heart rate variability can be an early indication of a future danger, like sudden cardiac arrest[12] or sepsis[13]. In the latter case, first HRV drops, before the symptom can be clinically detected. With hypertension, diabetes and arteriosclerotic processes, HRV-measuring is used for early detection of risks with people who have no other health problems (Wittling & Wittling 2012).

9. Heart Coherence and Heart Intelligence

The concept of heart coherence became popular through a US-institute named "HeartMath®". Its director is Doc Lew Childre and its team has published several books and texts (e.g. Childre, Martin & Beech 2000) to prove the strong power of the heart for improving health and mastering problems. Simple techniques were developed to increase and augment heart coherence. The main methods are breath relaxation and focusing the attention on the heart, connected with positive thoughts (Grimm 2015). However the relationships of coherence and resonance between breathing and heart rhythm, as described in the next chapter, are not included.

Although the findings of the heart research of Childre and his institute, which are spread with the registered trademarks *heartness* and *heart intelligence*, are presented as scientifically valid, we have to consider that the results have been achieved by the institute itself without outside proof from independent research institutions so far[14]. So there is extensive need for clarification to many of the claims brought up in this context.

Without any doubt, the recommended exercises are simple and helpful. It is always useful to pay attention to one's own organs, and the heart is of central importance. However, for achieving long term benefit for the health of our organism, lovingly conducted exercises in concentration are not enough in my opinion. We have to use a holistic approach to the autonomic regulatory circuits of our organism.

Coherent Breathing meets this claim, because it works with inner concentration as well as with mechanistic-dynamic regulation, which effectively influences the circulatory system. Double, mental and organic communication with autonomic processes is a benefit we can utilize by breathing consciously: Combining and harmonizing both approaches.

A coherent breather can add from heart intelligence the practice of focusing on positive thoughts and emotions, e.g. to let a feeling of gratitude come during Coherent Breathing and keeping the attention on the heart at the same time.

Important Points:

Coherence is a phenomenon in the physical world, in which materiel objects pursue harmony and order by themselves. The model of coherence can be transferred to the human organism.

Heart coherence means consistent changes of the heartbeat.

Heart rate variability signifies the ability of our heart to react appropriately to different demands.

The more variable the heartbeat is, the more flexible the reactive potential of heart and nervous system is.

By measuring heart rate variability, we can diagnose the state of health and the capability of sympathicus and parasympathicus.

Chapter 4 – The Breath-Heart Coherence

Now that we know and have the confirmation from science that a heart with a good rhythm is one of the most important fundaments of our health and well-being, the next question is what we can do to bring our heart into a good coherent mood and can keep it in this state.

So far, there are plenty of answers, from thinking loveable thoughts, spending reflective time in the forest to singing beautiful songs. Different forms of relaxing exercises and endurance trainings are also recommended. There are detailed plans for healthy nutrition and diet.

Yet the simplest key to our heart literally is so close: In close proximity to our heart are our lungs, which directly cooperate with the activity of the heart. With the work of our lungs, which is breathing, we have an excellent instrument for exerting influence on our heart. While the regulation of the heartbeat works autonomic, without influence from our will, we also can control our breathing voluntarily.

And this is our further topic: How do we have to use our breathing so that our heart achieves coherence and we come into coherence with our heart?

1. Lungs and Heart in Cooperation

First it is important to understand how breathing and heart cooperate. One thing is clear: The heart sends the venous blood, meaning poor in oxygen and rich in carbon-dioxide, from its right chamber to the lungs, in which the gas exchange takes place. Carbon-dioxide is released and fresh oxygen is taken up. This arterial blood then flows back to the left chamber to be distributed throughout the body via the arterial trunk.

The Pulmonary Circulation System

The lung circulation consists of the flow of the venous blood from the right atrium of the heart via the pulmonary trunk, which divides into the left and the right lung artery, to the lungs. The gas exchange transforms venous into arterial blood, which then flows back to the left atrium and from there into all areas of the body.

The pulmonary vascular resistance (PVR) of the pulmonary circulation is only a tenth of the total periphery resistance. This is why the blood pressure in the pulmonary circulation (20/8 mmHg) is considerably lower as in the main blood circulation (120/80 mmHg) (see fig. 8, p. 60).

The circulatory movements of the blood can be connected with the breathing movements, which will be discussed later. The breathing movements consist of widening the breathing space with the inhale and with diminishing the space with the exhale. This movement is mainly the task of the diaphragm, which can rise and fall 10 to 12 centimeters maximally. In addition, the intercostal muscles partici-pate in this movement by enlarging the chest space. When we breathe deeply, we use the whole volume of breathing (=vital capacity). With this volume, approximately 4.5 liters of air are exchanged.

Intercostal and Auxiliary Muscles for Breathing

Among the intercostal muscles, the internal and the external are the most important. The outer muscles contract in attunement with the inhalation, while the inner relax at the same time. Thus the ribs are drawn upwards and breathing has more space. We experience this process as widening of the breathing space, although it is caused by the contraction of the diaphragmatic and intercostal muscles.

The external intercostal muscles help in increasing the volume of the thorax by their contraction from front to back and from side to side. They are active in calm as well as in enforced inbreathing. They lift the ribs and stretch the transverse dimensions of the thorax.

The internal intercostals support the outbreath when it is done with force. They press the ribs to the inside and reduce the transverse dimensions of the thorax.

Besides the external and the internal intercostal muscles, there are the so-called intimate muscles situated between the external and the internal intercostals and these can support the exhalation.

We are also able to use the so-called expiratory auxiliary muscles (an example for this are the abdominal muscles) for consciously initiating exhalation. We need this with singing, talking or coughing. But also in the case of shortness of breath caused by asthma or other lung diseases like COPD, the conscious use of these muscles helps with the exhalation.

Using these auxiliary muscles for exhalation is called forced expiration. In this process, first the internal intercostal muscles contract. But also other auxiliary muscles can come into action. A special role in the context of forced exhalation is exerted by the so-called coughing muscle.

The Diaphragm as Pump

With inhalation, the diaphragm sinks downwards by contracting. Like in a pump, negative pressure is created, which lets the air stream in by itself. The relaxed diaphragm moves upwards, thus decreasing the volume of the breathing spaces and exhaling the air.

During this pumping movement the gas exchange happens: With inhalation, the air flows through the trachea and bronchial branches to the bronchioles, the tiny branches with the alveoli at their ends. Here the passing blood first releases its carbon-dioxide and then takes up the fresh oxygen. Enriched with oxygen, it flows back to the heart, which transports it as arterial blood into all areas of the body.

2. The Respiratory Sinusarrhythmia (RSA)

This monster of a word contains the sensitive attunement of heartbeat and breathing movement. During inhalation, the heartbeat increases and with exhalation, the heart slows down. So the heart frequency goes with the breathing rhythm, as it characteristically varies between inhalation and exhalation.

Figure 6 shows the complementarity of heart variability and heart frequency related to the breathing rhythm: With the heart beating quicker (lower curve), the R-R-intervals, i.e. the distances between the heartbeats (upper curve) decrease, so the variability is reduced. With inhalation, the heart beats faster and with exhalation slower, so that the curves reflect the breathing rhythm in each case. These records come from a measurement I undertook on myself.

5 Minutes Coherent Breathing (3 Breaths/Minute), R-R-Intervals

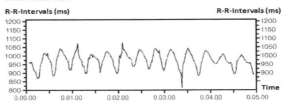

5 Minutes Coherent Breathing (3 Breaths/Minute), Heart Frequency

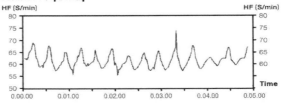

Fig. 6: Respiratory sinusarrhythmia

Here we come back to the influence of the autonomic nervous system. Roughly speaking, it shares its responsibility for the breathing process in the following ways: The sympathicus takes over the inhalation and cares for the acceleration of the heartbeat; the parasympathicus regulates exhalation and decelerates the heartbeat. Inhalation requires muscular work as the relevant breathing muscles have to contract. So the body needs more oxygen for more performance, and this is the responsibility of the sympathicus. Exhalation consists in resolving the tension, and this is the duty of the parasympathicus.

Respiratory sinusarrhythmia depends on the general state of the organism. The more relaxed, the clearer the arrhythmia is. So bigger differences between the heartbeat at inhalation and at exhalation signify a state of general relaxation. With increasing tension, these differences and with them heart rate variability, diminish. As soon as the sympathicus starts to dominate and drives back the parasympathicus, the coherence between heartbeat and breathing tends to get lost.

The Regulation of Respiratory Sinusarrhythmia

If you want to understand more about the regulation of the respiratory sinusarrhythmia, go on with reading here. If you are not so interested in the details, just skip this section.

In the brain stem, which is the oldest part of the brain, the centers regulating breathing and those regulating heart activity are closely connected. Researchers assume a central *respiratory generator* (Wittling & Wittling 2012, p. 121), which on one hand regulates the breathing frequency and on the other hand the speed of heartbeat through the parasympathicus. In this process, the parasympathical centers in the nucleus ambiguus of the brain stem sends impulses to the sinus node of the heart, which dampen its activity during exhalation. Thus the heart frequency is reduced, the heart beats slower. With inhalation, the influence of the parasympathicus gets inhibited, and this increases the speed of heartbeat. So in the case of breathing coherence, the respiratory center influences the heart circulatory center in the brain stem.

Besides the central regulation through the brain stem, where a central respiratory generator is assumed, there are other periphery mechanisms for influencing the breathing activity. We know that baroreceptors (mechanical measuring points of blood pressure at the vascular walls) and chemoreceptors stimulate the parasympathicus during outbreathing and reinforce its calming impact. On the other hand, stretching receptors in the lungs cause an inhibition of the parasympathicus during inhalation. These influences cause a further enhancement of the sinusarrhythmia.

The central respiratory generator not only influences the para-sympathicus but also the sympathicus. But this influence does not affect the sinus node directly, for it basically follows its own impulse program. This in turn sends contraction signals to the heart approximately 100 times a minute, except when getting an inhibitory signal from the parasympathicus sent by the neurotransmitter acetylcholine, which motivates the sinus node to reduce the heartbeat.

The amplitude of RSA, which is the amount of fluctuation between exhalation and inhalation indicates how strongly the parasympathicus can exert its inhibitory power. Consequently, the bigger the range of variability, the better the reduction of the sympathetic activity works – and the better the vagal brake works, cf. p. 29.

As explained in chapter 2.4 about the polyvagal theory, the efficiency of the vagal brake is crucial for the functioning of the *social engagement system*, respectively of the social interpersonal abilities like understanding, empathy, respect etc. Simplified, a weak performance of the parasympathicus in modulating the heartbeat complies with a low competence in social affairs. So we need a strong parasympathicus for maneuvering appropriately in the varying social fields.

3. The Valsalva Wave

This term was invented by Stephen Elliott and Dr. Bob Grove for the physical cooperation of heart and lung activity. The name is derived from Antonio Maria Valsalva, who lived as anatomist and surgeon from 1666 to 1723 in Italy. He initiated the Valsalva maneuver: it consists in exhaling deeply, holding the breath for 10 seconds and tensing up breathing and abdominal muscles. Thus more air pressure is generated in the respiratory ways. The exercise is used for pressure compensation in the middle ear as well as for checking the reflexes of the baroreceptors (which stabilizes the arterial blood pressure) and for normalizing the heartbeat when the heart is racing. Valsalva had noticed changes in the jugular vein, which corresponded to breathing, and was thus one of the first Western explorers of the relationship between breathing and blood circulation.

As above described, blood circulation and breathing meet in the lungs and ensure the supply with oxygen and the disposal of carbon-dioxide in the body. We can imagine the breathing as a pump, which creates a vacuum by contracting the diaphragm for the air to flow in. During relaxation the diaphragm moves upwards and presses out the exhalation air rich of carbon-dioxide. Additionally, the diaphragm can exert a pumping activity effecting the blood circulation: With the influx of air at the inhalation, the venous blood from the right chamber of the heart comes into the lungs via the lung arteries. With the counter-movement during exhalation, the oxygen enriched blood is pumped back to the heart's left chamber, from where it is

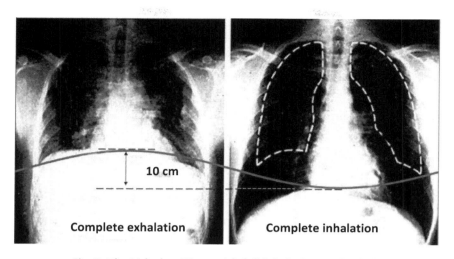

10 cm

Complete exhalation | Complete inhalation

Fig. 7: The Valsalva-Wave with full inhalation and exhalation
(reprinted by kind permission of Stephen Elliott)

distributed throughout the organism. The negative pressure effective during inhalation not only draws the air but also the blood into the lungs. The positive pressure at exhalation then pumps the blood back to the heart.

The changing pressure conditions in the blood circulation, which get reinforced by Coherent Breathing movements, turn the rib-cage into a pump, the thorax pump. It supports the heart and the vascular system with the dynamics of blood flow and provides a rhythm streaming as a wavelike movement throughout the whole upper body.

The term Valsalva-wave describes the whole phenomenon of the rise and fall of pressure in the bloodstream, initiated by the nervous system. It comprises the arterial pressure wave as well as its venous counterpart, connected with the increase and decrease of heart frequency. The breathing movement acts as central rhythm generator, which initiates and maintains the wave.

4. Diaphragm and Blood Pressure

So the Valsalva-wave is stimulated by the diaphragm, when it supports the heart in its pumping activity. This only works when there is a breathing rhythm, which fits into the time-wise necessities of the blood streams between heart and lungs. When the breathing is too fast, there is not enough time for the blood to flow in, respectively for the blood to flow back into the heart. In this case, the heart has to do the pumping on its own. When the breathing is too slow, the same happens.

Elliott talks about three pumps for the circulatory system: Heart, arterial trunk with its contracting movements, and the diaphragm. When all of them work in a shared rhythm, the conditions for coherence are created. In this case breathing acts as main impulse generator synchronizing heart and blood circulation. This consonance is called Valsalva-wave (personal sharing).

The volume of blood exchange depends on the depth of the breathing movement, which is equivalent to the respiratory volume. In the ideal case, the volume is used optimally by the blood vessels: Not too much and not too little blood can flow into the lungs and out of them. During inhalation the venous flow is accentuated and during

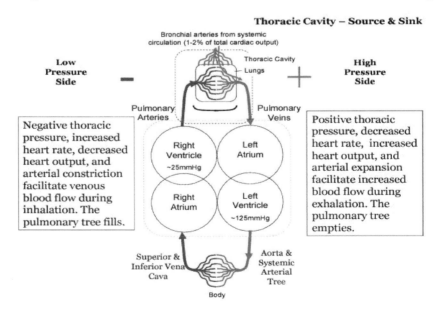

Fig. 8: The Valsalva-Wave (reprinted by kind permission of Stephen Elliott)

exhalation the arterial flow is accentuated. During inhalation, with the rise of the heartbeat, blood pressure sinks; during exhalation, it rises and the heartbeat slows down. Thus a wave of circulation is created, rising in the arterial trunk with exhalation and sinking with the inhalation. The opposite happens in the venous trunk: the pressure wave rises with inhalation and falls with exhalation. This wave is supported by vascular contractions: The vessels dilate with the rise of blood pressure during exhalation and constrict with its fall (Lehrer & Gevirtz 2014, p. 4).

Blood expelled with exhalation from the lungs flows via the lung veins to the right chamber of the heart, which enhances its pressure and thus distributes the blood via the arteries in the whole body. The baroreceptors in the arteries measure the pressure conditions and signal to the autonomic nervous system to accelerate or decelerate the heartbeat correspondingly. So the heart frequency rises and falls in opposition to the blood wave initiated by breathing.

As the lungs need the same amount of time for filling and emptying, it is important that the breathing rhythm is even, that the time for inhalation is equal to the time for exhalation.

Optimal breathing for the cooperation of diaphragmatic breathing and heart activity is then called Coherent Breathing. It uses a breathing rhythm between roughly three and six breaths per minute, so it is relatively slow. Inbreaths and outbreaths have the same length, each between five or ten seconds. Details and instructions for practice follow in the next chapter.

The interconnections between heartbeat and blood pressure were discovered by the Russian researcher Evgeny Vaschillo in the nineteen-eighties, who wanted to improve the performance of top athletes. According to Vaschillo, there is a resonance frequency, at which the oscillations of heartbeat and blood pressure are out of phase by 180 degrees: Heartrate is highest, when blood pressure is reduced and vice versa approximately six seconds later. With this frequency, the pressure sensitive baroreceptors of the aorta and the carotid are maximally stimulated. By the stimulation of these receptors, signals go the brain stem via the vagus nerve and influence the brain functions.

5. Valsalva Wave and Brain

As the Valsalva-wave includes the whole body through the blood circulation and is measurable at different spots, it is very likely that it also acts on the brain: The cerebrospinal fluidity (CSF) takes care of cleaning the brain from debris similar to the lymphatic system in the rest of the body. Among others, the peptide amyloid-beta gets disposed of, which plays a role in the development of Alzheimer's. CSF is kept in movement by the pressure difference in the circulatory system.

This cleansing process best works during sleep. This is one of the reasons why humans need sleep. Humans sleep horizontally so that the hydrostatic pressure effects of gravity on the whole body can normalize. As we breathe more evenly during sleep, Elliott thinks that CSF-transport works better during sleep. When the CSF-transport is a question of pressure distribution, it should increase during Coherent Breathing. During sleep, the inertia of blood in the head is equal to the one in the feet. This is a reason that optimal breathing is possible in the lying position.

Important Points:

By regulating our breathing, we can increase our heart rate variability and influence heart coherence.

The cooperation of breathing, heart and autonomic nervous system expresses the respiratory sinusarrhythmia: The heart frequency rises during inhalation and falls during exhalation.

The breathing movement, mainly supported by the diaphragm, can support the pumping activity of the heart, thus creating the Valsalva-Wave.

Through this wave, venous blood is drawn to the lungs during inhalation, while the oxygen enriched blood is distributed in the organism during exhalation.

Presumably the Valsalva-Wave also acts to stimulate and cleanse the brain.

Chapter 5 – Coherent Breathing

1. The History

The phenomenon of respiratory sinusarrhythmia in connection with arterial blood pressure was already an important subject of medical research at the beginning of the 20th century. After that, the scientific community lost interest in these findings. Only in the nineties of the twentieth century, the fast rise of HRV measurement and research initiated a renaissance of the interest in the relationship between breathing and heart activity. Thousands of scientific publications on heart rate variability have been produced in the last decades, and its measurement has become an important part of medical routine checkups, finding its way into leisure as well as professional sports.

However there are hardly any studies on the role breathing has on influencing the variability of the heartbeat, in the contrary, some studies suppose that there is no possibility of influencing the activity of the heart by changing the breathing. This can have its cause that the experiments were conducted with breathing frequencies faster than those recommended in Coherent Breathing.

The discovery of Coherent Breathing is closely connected with Stephen Elliott who had previously studied yoga in Yoga in China and India. The story starts in 2001, when Elliott visited the integrative neurotherapist Dee Edmundson in Plano (USA) with his 11-years old son, who suffered from attention deficit syndrome, for a biofeedback session. She introduced Elliott to the model of heart rate variability, which had been hardly known at that time. This biofeedback session was about coordinating breathing with one's own heart rhythm shown by the biofeedback device.

Elliott was excited about the connections between breathing and heart rhythm, which could be visualized by the measures. He had already experimented with measuring the brain waves in meditation at that time and discovered that he could reach the desired brain frequency state quickly by using the breathing rhythm from the biofeedback measuring.

So it became clear that there should be a certain breathing rhythm, which could bring other rhythms of the body in unison, another form of coherence, and soon after that Coherent Breathing was invented.

In 2008, Elliott and Edmundson published the book „Coherent Breathing. The Definitive Method", in which some smaller research projects were also described. Elliott and Edmundson write: "Over and above our personal experience, Coherent Breathing is presently employed by 100s of health care professionals and 1000s of individual practitioners in 9 nations, where many are also observing or personally experiencing dramatic enhancements in health, well-being, and performance." (Elliott & Edmundson 2008, p. 8)

In 2012, the book „The Healing Power of the Breath" by Brown and Gerberg was published with a lot of case studies from clinical practice and impressive reports from working with big groups after catastrophes in various crisis zones. It could be proven that con-sequences of trauma and posttraumatic stress disorders can be relieved with exercises from Coherent Breathing.

Elliott and Edmundson write, that despite thousands of studies on observing and analyzing HRV "there is surprisingly little written as to 'what the heart rate variability phenomenon actually is'". (Elliott & Edmundson 2008, p. 8)

However by better understanding the physiology of breathing and its regulation by the autonomic nervous system there is progress in this area: The discovery of the thoracic pump explains the connection between breathing, autonomic nervous system and arterial blood pressure (respiratory arterial pressure = RAP). The RAP wave exists as long as we breathe coherently. A missing or weakened RAP wave has negative effects on our health and probably even on our life expectancy, as the autonomic nervous system needs the RAP wave for maintaining homeostasis. In the neutral state, the diaphragm con-tributes a lot to the movements of the blood and relieves the heart and vascular system from the burden of having to generate and maintain the whole blood pressure and blood movement throughout the body.

When the RAP wave works, the ANS swings with every in- and outbreath: With the inbreath, it goes towards the sympathicus, with the outbreath towards the parasympathicus. In sum this results in a balanced nervous system. These wavelike oscillations can be detected and measured in various physical functions: Blood flow, heartbeat, arterial pressure, skin conductivity, brain waves and muscular tension. For these relationships, Elliott created together with Dr. Bob Grove the term "Valsalva-Wave™". Stephen Elliott holds numerous patents for methods and devices supporting Coherent Breathing.

2. The Method of Coherent Breathing

This is an overview over the **basic rules of Coherent Breathing**:

1. Breathing takes equal time for inhalation and exhalation. There are no pauses between the breaths.

2. Breathing follows a steady and consistent rhythm during practice. Recommended are three to six breaths per minute. This corresponds to 10 to 5 seconds per inbreath and 10 to 5 seconds per outbreath.

3. Breathing with a comfortable middle depth. As the diaphragm moves a distance of 10 to 12 cm distance between the maximally tensed and maximally relaxed state, Coherent Breathing recommends a diaphragm movement of 4 to 6 cm. The maximal breathing volume should be used to ca. 50%.

4. The outbreath is relaxed. While a certain degree of muscular tension is required for inhaling, which needs to contract diaphragm and intercostal muscles, exhalation happens by resolving this tension.

3. The Elements of Coherent Breathing

Here comes a detailed explanation of the tenets of Coherent Breathing:

1. Equal Length of Inhalation an Exhalation

The aim of Coherent Breathing is synchronicity of breathing, heartbeat and blood circulation. When breathing in, blood is drawn from the heart to the lungs, when breathing out, blood leaves the lungs. At the same time, blood is distributed throughout the body respectively collected and drawn back. For both processes, the same amount of time is needed, and when this time is provided, the whole system is in optimal balance. The result of breath-heart-circulation-coherence in terms of the Valsalva wave can only be achieved when the duration of inhalation equals the duration of exhalation.

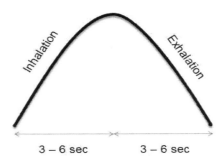

Fig. 9: Regular breathing = equal duration of inhalation and exhalation

To get a sense for this regularity of breathing, it is useful to start with time-keeping devices. We can follow the second hand on a watch or an electronic device. Even more useful are apps available for smartphones, where the breathing rhythm can be timed up to a tenth of a second, and gives acoustic signals. Thus the eyes do not have to do the controlling by following the second hand, but convenient sounds help us to switch from inbreath to outbreath. Listening is better for relaxation than visual observation and allows us to close our eyes. Digital devices provide exact impulses with respect to consistency.

After having worked with an external signal generator, we acquire a sense for regularity and also for frequency. Henceforth, we also can practice Coherent Breathing without external devices. Now we have the freedom to practice virtually everywhere. We do not need a totally exact signal from outside, and this is beneficial for us also in the sense that our body does not know digital accuracy and con-sequently reacts defensively when confronted with it. In the free flow of breathing with approximate exactness, we best fulfill the demands of the first basic rule. Still it is recommended to use a time-keeper on and off during free practice to check whether the timing is still in the coherent frame.

Prolonged Exhalation?

There are various breathing techniques with prolonged exhalation that are used to deepen the effect of relaxation, especially when there is a lot of tension. E.g. there is the 2-4-2-breathing: breathing in at two counts, breathing out on four and pausing for two counts. By this or similar exercises the vagal brake can be activated rather quickly, which reduces the activity of the sympathicus and calms down the nervous system. In extending the exhalation, the parasympathicus gets more time to become active. This becomes noticeable via a subjective feeling of pleasant relaxation that many people have when stretching the outbreath without pressure for the next inbreath. It has also been found that people with a lot of experience in meditation often spontaneously develop a habit of prolonging the outbreath.

In the Sufi tradition, there are some breathing exercises, in which the exhalation is prolonged considerably, sometimes in the ratio of 1:4 or even 1:8. Yet there are other teachings in this tradition recommending breathing in and out like the pendulum of a watch: "When our breathing goes rhythmically, everything is fine."

We have to consider that, as far as we currently know, heart rate variability drops when the outbreath is stretched. This would be a confirmation of the following assumption: Longer exhalation reduces acute stress, which leads to a feeling of relief. However the parasympathicus will not be strengthened long-lastingly, as there will be no heart coherence, no synchronicity of the pumping activity of the heart with breathing. Although the vagal brake gets activated quickly, but not trained, no Valsalva wave is generated. The wavelike effect of breathing on the blood circulation is absent in this instance, for which it needs equal lengths of inbreath and outbreath. All we have is a relaxing effect for the moment.

Elliott has formulated the following hypothesis: By delaying the inhalation, which causes a delay of the negative pressure in the thoracic cave, the right heart chamber has to work faster for keeping up the flow in the venous system. When this flow cannot be maintained, the pressure in the arterial system will grow.

However breathing exercises working with prolonged exhalation can be very beneficial for calming down from an acute state of over tension. We can use such exercises for entering into the Coherent Breathing rhythm. See the recommendations in chapter 6.6, p. 85 ff.

2. Frequency (Speed)

Measurements of respiratory sinusarrhythmia as well as in other parameters of HRV have shown that the range of the heart frequency is significantly stronger in the area between 3 and 6 breaths per minute. This means that we can produce the favorable values of heart rate variability with this breathing rhythm in regards to the amount (the amplitude of RSA) as well as the regularity. When we breathe quicker than the optimal resonance frequency (some others mention 5 breaths as upper limit, others 7), the sympathicus comes too strongly into play. Thus breathing gets involved in the stress system, with an increasing tendency: The quicker the more sympathetic dominance, the more stress. Heart rate variability successively decreases with the rate of shifting to the sympathetic area, which is indicated by a breathing frequency accelerating beyond 5, 6 or 7 breaths per minute.

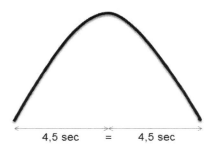

4,5 sec   =   4,5 sec

Fig. 10: Example for a Coherent Breathing frequency

Below 3 breaths per minute, in the area of extreme slow breathing, the regularity of RSA, the differences of the heartbeat frequency between inbreath and outbreath, all become more irregular and chaotic. When the breaths are overstretched, although we can do this deliberately, an inner pressure seems to join in, which leaves little space for relaxation. So the sympathicus will start to take of the control and reduces the intended improvement of the parasympathetic power and of heart rate variability. However there is not enough research information or studies to this subject, to my knowledge.

Which breathing frequency within the favorable range for HRV should we choose for our practice? A parameter is the physical size of the lungs in connection with height. Taller people have bigger lungs and hearts, and the blood circulation covers longer distances in their blood circulation system. They will find breathing with slow frequencies between five and three breaths per minute more appropriate. Smaller persons will feel more at ease in the frequency range of five or six breaths per minute. With children, this value is usually between seven and ten breaths per minute.

For some persons (especially those with habitual short breathing), who start practicing with Coherent Breathing, the regular frequency of five to six breaths per minute can only be managed under pressure and strain. They have to stretch their breathing so far beyond the usual range that it can only be done with effort and trouble.

As any kind of stress and pressure is counter-productive for practicing breath coherence, it is recommended to start breathing with a frequency, which can be kept up conveniently over a time of some minutes, even if it is around 10 or 12 breaths per minute. In any case, the aim would be to prolong the breathing step by step and decelerate the breaths until the recommended range of frequency is reached.

Practicing successively decelerating the breathing, in connection with a regular pattern, is as such an important step to reduce inner stress. This is because, when we cannot breathe slowly, chronified stress is activated, and this means that the body is constantly oversteered by the sympathicus. Every step closer to the optimal frequency calms our autonomic nervous system back to its equilibrium.

Individual Resonance Frequency

Some evaluation programs of HRV measurements calculate the exact individual value of resonance. Someone can have the optimal breathing rhythm at 4.7 breaths per minute. Stephen Elliott calls this value the resonance frequency, which can be measured by a specific device for recording the Valsalva wave. The patented instrument uses an optic plethysmograph, which measures the blood flow via a finger or ear clip. With special software, the measurement can be evaluated for stating the individual frequency of resonance, although there is still no assured knowledge about this subject. But a sufficient number of individual measurements have shown that heart rate variability is higher, when one breathes with the exact individual resonance frequency.

This is an explanation based on the current state of knowledge. When we breathe with equal duration of inbreath and outbreath, breathing dominates the heartbeat. When breathing is resonant, it has the biggest impact on the heartbeat, because the latter will follow the breathing. Theoretically, resonant breathing is the frequency in which the heart-circulatory system oscillates naturally. Every person has an individual resonance frequency strongly correlating with height. In order to figure that out, according to Stephen Elliott, heart rate variability is not sufficient as the only parameter, although later in this section we find a measuring technique developed by Evgeny Vaschillo, by which this individual resonance value can be defined with the RMSSD value.

We have to know what the blood does and what the heart does – in relation to the breathing frequency. When we breathe at a speed close to our individual resonance rate, the heart will tune in to this rhythm even if the breathing frequency does not match the resonance frequency exactly. The autonomic nervous system will hang on to breathing, similar to the classical physical resonance experiment where weaker pendulums follow the stronger ones. This shows the "power" of breathing over inner coherence. When we understand that the HRV cycle is the autonomic answer to our breathing, we can breathe in synchronicity with it. Thus we close a positive feedback loop between our mind, our nervous system and our breathing. An oscillation is formed, which generates a sinus wave in the whole circulatory system and beyond (Elliott 2016, p. 4 – 7).

Yet for efficient practice, the exact individual resonance frequency is not necessarily required. The special benefit of the resonance frequency lies in creating the optimal gain when practicing Coherent

Breathing. Those who want to investigate deeper and experiment with their own breathing, can purchase Elliott's special plethysmograph on the site of Coherence LLC or carry out the following practice and measurement series according to Evgeny Vaschillo:

You breathe to each of the following frequencies for one minute: 8, 7, 6, 5 and 4 rpm (respirations per minute). Then you compare the RMSSD values: With which frequency the outcome is highest? If the best result is e.g. with 5, you define another five ranges around 5: e.g. 6.0, 5.5, 5.0, 4.5, 4.0 rpm. Again, the maximum is determined, e.g. 4.5. For fine-tuning, again five ranges are defined, e.g. 4.7, 4.6, 4.5, 4.4, 4.3. The maximal value from this measurement is your individual coherent resonance frequency, e.g. 4.6.

Like other practitioners I consider practicing within the recom-mended range of three to five or six breaths to be sufficient for the beginner. You can use a device for keeping time, until you obtain enough feeling for the exercise that you can practice freely with your own convenient rhythm. Thus you gain more and more self-competence. Step by step, you acquire inner safety to choose the appropriate breathing rhythm. You then know from experience when you are within the frequency range of your coherent resonance and do not have to control it by external devices. From time to time, you will check whether your practice frequency matches the goal area, but more and more you learn to trust your feeling. By this, you develop autonomy in practice and an inner competence to be able to evaluate your inner state and its requirements.

As in many other areas of life, there are persons, who are satisfied with good results and others who want to investigate further. It is up to you as reader, which way you want to choose to practice. This book offers as much encouragement and motivation for both styles of practice so that by reading and by applying the exercises it will become clear, what your personal way will be.

3. Depth (the Volume)

When the breathing is too shallow, the diaphragm is not engaged. This is the cause of many breathing disorders. The auxiliary breathing muscles take over the work necessary for breathing and not the diaphragm, our original and most important breathing muscle. With this misuse, we overstrain the auxiliary muscles with tensions in the shoulder and neck area as unpleasant consequence, often ending with a headache or migraine.

Furthermore, when we just use the diaphragm minimally, e.g. by just allowing an up and down movement of one to two centimeters, we limit the space for the exchange movements of heart and lungs, and less blood will be sucked in and expelled out of the lungs. In this case, the diaphragm supports the heart in its pumping activity only very little.

On the other hand, according to the available evidence, 50 – 60 % of the maximally possible breathing volume is sufficient for practicing Coherent Breathing. We need the full capacity for breathing in conditions of performance in sports, in strenuous work, in singing or playing a woodwind instrument. Practice should be done under relaxed conditions and not with the maximal volume, which would again create a stress factor. As explained right afterwards, the out-breathing should be relaxed. Thus we remain in an area of pleasantly deepened breathing, of an expanded comfort zone and do not experiment with stretching and contracting the breathing spaces to a maximum. In the middle segment of the potential volume, we can let the exhalation flow out free from any control.

Moreover, people with little experience of breathing practices will gradually expand the breath volume so that slowly the range of pleasantly deepened breathing increases. This means in scientific terms, that the total surface of the alveoli expands, which intensifies and improves the gas exchange.

How can you find the right breathing depth? Take a few full breaths by opening up your breathing spaces in chest, belly and lower back as much as possible. So you get a sense of your maximal breath volume (your vital capacity) and for the maximal movement of your diaphragm during breathing. Now find a middle depth between shallow and maximal breathing. This volume will be larger than your normal daily breathing and smaller than your vital capacity. You will notice that your diaphragm will move about a handwidth up and down. You will notice the movement of your abdominal wall, both visually and internally.

4. Relaxation of the Exhalation

Our breathing is kept going by muscular activity. Muscles have basically two directions of movement: contraction and letting go of contraction. The first is work, the latter interruption of work, the first requires energy, the latter does not.

We notice this difference when making a fist. We need energy and we feel it. When opening the fist, we end the exertion of force and the fist opens by itself. Of course, we can open the fist with force and will immediately notice the difference between contraction and relaxation. In breathing, this principle can be found in the contraction for inhalation and the relaxation for exhalation. When we inhale, the muscles involved in breathing contract and create a vacuum, with exhalation, the contraction reduces, and the air flows out according to the amount of decreasing contraction. So the process of exhalation principally works by muscular relaxation. Yet for many people, relaxed exhalation is easier said than done. We are used to exhaling with pressure (possibly only slight) and thus we apply force and energy in the process, which naturally works without it. We breathe like forcefully opening a fist.

And by this, we have, generally speaking, implemented stress into our exhalation. For this means on the level of the nervous system that the sympathicus, which is in charge of processes of contraction, takes part in inbreathing as well as outbreathing. Thus the whole organism comes into a detrimental and potentially unhealthy imbalance, as the parasympathetic part is strongly reduced.

So it is of crucial importance to find the way to relax the exhale. This principle underlies many schools of breathwork, so I feel tempted to change the 2500 years old saying of Confucius: "What has to be taught first is the breath" to something more relevant for our contemporary world: "What has to be taught first is the relaxed exhale."

Relaxing the outbreathing means strengthening the parasympathicus and this is the key for implementing the breath-heart-coherence. Without equality for the parasympathicus in the breathing process, there is no coherence. Yet relaxation cannot be "made" or "done" as it is basically non-action. Normally, our bodies do not exhale by doing something, by being active, but by interrupting action until with the next inhalation action is possible and necessary.

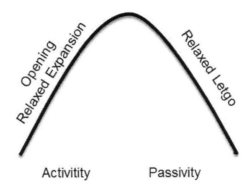

Fig. 11: Relaxed exhalation

So how can we learn to exhale in a relaxed way? There is a big and a small path for this task. The big path leads back to life events, which manifested as tensions in the breathing muscles. These tensions contain fears, which can be resolved in gentle therapeutic work. It is the path of integrative or psychotherapeutic breathwork. It requires not just the necessary time invested, but also the inner willingness to face the problems of one's life in order to free oneself from the imprinted inhibitions and detriments with long lasting effect. More to this in chapter 10 and 11.

The small path consists of careful self-study and patient practice, in which one can work with the imagination of relaxation: I imagine dropping everything with the exhale, becoming light and free, only letting gravity work.

However some cannot imagine how relaxed exhalation might feel like. Here a variation of the exercise with the fist can help: Lift a hand with inhalation with tension and let it fall with exhalation, without any force. So inhalation happens with force and strength like lifting the arm, and exhalation with powerlessness, as if gravity would pull everything down without our participation.

Learning relaxed exhalation is a gradual process, leading to success only by practice, and it is a necessary process, as tensed exhalation is always a sign for chronic stress patterns. In the tensed exhalation, the diaphragm takes part by exerting pressure on the abdominal area and also the internal intercostal muscles, and this process is directed by the sympathicus, so it has no relaxing effect.

The training process towards relaxing the exhalation, which we go through with patient practice, is helpful for many factors of stress. For example, people with sleep problems (problems with falling asleep and sleeping through) can find better, deeper and more restorative sleep, when they have trained relaxed exhalation.

A woman reported that after learning Coherent Breathing in a seminar, she slept well the following night for the first time in many years. She was very happy about it. She used Coherent Breathing to help her falling asleep and whenever she woke up during the night, she quickly managed to fall back asleep again. A few months later she told me that on the whole, the improvement had been stable, but now and then, when she had a conversation on the phone with her daughter, who lived abroad, she found it hard to sleep well. A trauma she had experienced with her daughter a long time ago has not lost completely its grip on her. Obviously, a longer period of time was needed overall for the parasympathicus to acquire enough competence and power to cope with this strongly stress-loaded memory.

Inhalation in Coherent Breathing is not done by accident, but as conscious and loose expansion connected the idea of relaxation. So the inbreath is not taken in a hectic and pressured way but lightly and easily. Imagining opening the breathing space can help so that the air can flow in by itself, without effort. Actually we do not suck in the air, rather the activity lies just in opening up a hollow space by contracting the breathing muscles. As a vacuum, this space attracts the air to flow in by itself. So during breathing in, the physiological relaxation of breathing out is mentally prepared, which enhances the effect of relaxation.

5. Evenness and Consistency

Phase, frequency and depth (volume) are maintained during the cycle of practice. In this way, the body gets increasingly attuned to coherence. The nervous system and the other physical systems stimulated by it, adjust to this basic rhythm and vibrate in accordance with it and among them. Thus, a persistently and consistently un-dulating wave is generated, which ultimately includes the whole body and mind.

6. The Importance of Nose Breathing

In Coherent Breathing we use the nose for inhalation and exhalation. The breath should generally flow through the nose, our main breathing channel. We should only breathe through the mouth, when we have a special purpose for it, giving ourselves the per-mission to breathe through the mouth under certain exceptional conditions only. Afterwards, we return to the normal state, to nose breathing. In the practice of Coherent Breathing, there is no purpose for mouth breathing, so we breathe only through the nose.

There are two main occasions for mouth breathing. The main one is connected with the breathing volume: We can inhale a lot more air through the mouth. So when we need a lot of air and oxygen e.g. for strenuous work or sportive activities, we have to breathe through the mouth. The second occasion is due to the fact that we only can speak and sing with open mouth and air streaming out.

Excursus: Nitrogen and Nose Breathing

Nitrogen monoxide (NO) is a gas we know as environmental polluter and originator of summer smog in cities. It is generated in combustion and occurs in strong concentration inter alia in cigarette smoke and exhaust gases of cars. So it was sensational, when it could be proven that NO is also formed in the human body and fulfils important functions there.

For this discovery, three US researchers were awarded the 1998 Nobel Prize for medicine. They could prove that nitrogen fulfils a role for regulating the tonus of the blood vessels that is for the relaxation of the blood circulation. NO is constantly produced in the walls of the vessels. The small gas molecules expand the vessels for improving the circulation. The gas is also involved in the functioning of the nervous system and is able to destroy bacteria and viruses.

Meanwhile we know that big amounts of nitrogen are formed in human sinuses. The sinuses are in connection with the nasal cavity through small openings, and this means that the level of NO is also very high in the nasal air[15].

With inhalation, nitrogen goes to the lungs with the air, but only, when we breathe through the nose. As NO is expanding vessels, the vessels, which get in contact with the alveoli, expand. This means that a higher amount of blood passing through the alveoli can be enriched with oxygen.

Comparing nasal breathing with mouth breathing, it could be demonstrated that nose breathing leads to 10-15% more oxygen binding in the blood. When NO is added to mouth breathing from a gas container, the same effect applies. So it is the nitrogen in the nasal air causing the beneficial effects.

In other experiments patients were intubated, i.e. they got a tube from a lung ventilator leading directly down the breathing ways. So their noses could not take part in breathing. A simple pumping system was applied, sucking air from one nostril, and this air then was added to the air coming from the ventilator. This procedure increased blood oxidation by 10 to 20 % (cf. McKeown 2011).

These discoveries point at a new principle, according to which an efficient substance, NO, is formed by the body in the sinuses and transported onwards with the inhaled air to cause effects in another part of the body, the lungs. Thus nitrogen acts as an air transported mediator in the human airways.

When looking into the world of animals, only the monkeys and elephants have NO in their noses. Other species do not have this system. Researchers think that monkeys and humans need this system to optimize oxygen binding required for upright walking.

Additionally, it has been proven that humming stimulates the production of NO and spreads it better among the sinuses. A study in

„*The European Respiratory Journal*"[16] came to the conclusion: Several phases of humming during the day reduce the risk for sinus problems. A continuous stream of air between the sinuses in the head not inhibited by mucus protects against inflammations, sinusitis and rhinitis.

The emphasis on consistent nose breathing we know from Buteyko-breathing, which will be discussed more in chapter 8. Training and prolonging the Buteyko control pause (holding the breath with closed nose up to the point of the inhalation reflex) as well as exercises for opening a clogged nose serve for increasing the formation of the gas.

Nasal breathing is also important for health prevention, because less allergens and viruses get to the lower breathing ways. Each breath also brings NO into the lower breathing areas, where it causes vasodilatory and anti-inflammatory effects.

Important Points:

Coherent has the following basic tenets:

- In- and outbreaths are equal in length.
- The rhythm is between three and six breaths per minute.
- The breathing volume is of middle depth.
- Exhalation is relaxed.
- Breathing goes through the nose only.

By breathing through the nose, we provide the body with more nitrogen, a gas with vasodilatory and anti-inflammatory effects.

The determination of the personal resonance frequency requires more detailed measurement and can improve the training benefit.

Chapter 6 – Practicing Coherent Breathing

Learning Coherent Breathing requires time. Let us not forget that our vegetative nervous system was installed in the early prenatal phase, developed its mode of functioning during this time and kept it essentially during the course of our lives, even when it is out of balance and chronically overstressed. When we start to re-educate it, we need consistency and patience. Changes come slow and will be noticed slowly. This can need weeks or months. But success is inevitable, for as the nervous system initially learned without conscious participation to optimally cope with prevailing environmental conditions, it now learns to align with new situations with our conscious support much better.

With training we mainly empower the parasympathicus, so it can become an equivalent partner and fully perform its role as regulator of the sympathicus. Thus we lay the foundations for balancing the nervous system, which enables the inner systems to work optimally. This is where success will initially occur: In the regulatory circuits, in which everything that has been proven to be beneficial and energy saving, a positive feedback loop is established, which strengthens the training effect.

The autonomic nervous system does not learn in leaps but continuously. So it is unlikely that we perceive sudden changes during practice. Rather the restructuring process is ongoing and happens gradually like the slow swelling of a river or the increase of wind. As our nervous system "strives" towards acting in its genuine form, we only work against unfavorable habits in our practice, habits that have been established in the course of life, and not against the basic current of our organism. It is precisely this original way of functioning designed by nature that we want to restore with united forces: With the help of our highly developed cognitive functions, which provide knowledge, motivation, commitment and consistency for our practice and with the help of the wisdom of our autonomic processes, which seek the way to their simplest and most effective mode of functioning by themselves as soon as we grant the space for that.

1. Regaining the Original Mode

Coherent Breathing is the way, which leads heart, lungs and blood circulation to their best way of cooperation as designed by nature. So further vegetative systems get supported: The lymphatic system, which is kept moving by blood circulation and breathing, digestion, which can work best with the rhythm of diaphragmatic breathing and the dominance of the parasympathicus, the immune system, which also needs a strong parasympathicus, and the brain, which gets cleansed and detoxified by the Valsalva Wave and can better balance its evolutionary older and younger functions with a balanced auto-nomic nervous system and thus find an optimal coordination.

The exercises presented here do not claim to be the "right" or "optimal" way of breathing for all situations in life. So we do not need to put ourselves under pressure by thinking that we should breathe coherently all the time from now on. Also with other practices and methods the goal is not to use them all around the clock. Practices serve life, not the other way round. Breathing exercises serve the breath in life, in all aspects.

Practice changes breathing so that a slower and more balanced form of breathing can be taken over by unconscious breathing. The learning processes in the brain stem, where breathing is regulated, happen through conditioning that occurs through focused, concen-trated, enduring but not uninterrupted repetition.

The way we breathe "normally", that is what we consider as our common breathing pattern to be, is the result of a learning process containing the sum of significant experiences we have collected in the course of our lives with breathing as steady companion – physio-logical and psycho-emotional experiences. The habits that make up our way of living are part of that, e.g. the amount of motion, sports, etc. as well as our ways of reacting emotionally with their impact on the level of stress: Do we react quickly and intensely to unexpected changes in the outer reality or can we stay calm under most circumstances?

When considering the formation of such habits we can assume that earlier experiences have a greater impact on us than later ones. The same is true for regular ways of behavior and their impact, over and above those that rarely occur. Lastly, the same goes for emotionally more intense events as opposed to harmless ones.

Practicing Coherent Breathing motivates the brain and nervous system to form new reflexes and build on that to create new structures and patterns. The more often and regular the exercises happen, the more effective the learning process is. Such processes are solidified by repetition and feedback. Relief from stress as a result of the conscious regulation of breathing, activation of the parasympathicus by relaxing the exhale and the support of the circulatory system by breathing coherently are factors, which positively reflect back to the learning processes in the brain stem. So we can assume that the desired improvement of the breathing function will flow more and more into our daily way of breathing so that we start to breathe more regularly and in a more relaxed fashion with middle depth even in situations where we do not pay attention to our breathing.

2. Practice and Resistance

Additionally the positive effects of Coherent Breathing practices on heart rate variability indicate that the whole organism, mediated over the autonomic nervous system, acquires more flexibility, which indicates the ability to react appropriately to the demands of different situations and events. This includes the important ability to find our way back to the recreative mode as fast as possible after stressful experiences. Stress in the right dose is not detrimental as such, rather it is beneficial for our health; yet when after a stress reaction the regulation back to relaxation does not work, the basic systems of our organism come into imbalance and this is the way to turn dysfunctional habits of inner regulation into chronic ones.

Practicing Coherent Breathing involves a limitation in itself, which we should keep in mind. When we focus on the accuracy of breathing, we apply a certain amount of cognitive strain, which restricts HRV. A study[17] confirms that simple exercises in mindfulness done with the instruction to pay attention only to the present experience require less control and less active concentration. As a consequence, the parasympathicus improves better than with guided and controlled breathing exercises.

However we know from experience that practicing Coherent Breathing tends toward creating more lightness and ease with time by letting go of diligent concentration on "right/wrong" or "exact/sloppy". Instead of engaging in control by thinking, the feeling of accuracy comes from inside. The practicing person feels as soon as she has found a good breathing rhythm without having to supervise the timing with a measuring device constantly.

In the beginning it can be helpful to dismiss the word "control" as soon as it arises. When practicing with acoustic signals guiding the breathing with rising and falling sounds, we can try to merge with the sounds in our imagination.

We have the opportunity to subtly mix stress into each exercise: "I have to practice as much as possible or follow all the rules exactly, otherwise I will not get to the desired results." More important than sticking to the rules is a relaxed and meditative attitude and the inner trust that we are on the right path and that this path is wider than rigid rules. Flexibility means also that we can switch from more rigid units of practice to more comfortable ones.

We also should keep in mind that it is not about constantly maximizing our heart rate variability, as with this aim we would not have any power for sports, could not do strenuous jobs, lift heavy goods or watch a horror movie.

But we should not lose sight of the principle: After either physi-cally or emotionally strenuous and burdening experiences, which shift our inner conditions towards sympathetic bias, we have to indulge in a sufficient phase of regeneration for our HRV and emo-tional status to regain balance. To lead a flexible life with challenges on different levels and various spaces for recreation is the best guarantee for the variability of our inner governance.

There is a resistance against any exercise: It is not necessarily manageable to sit down on a regular basis to calm down the breathing for a few minutes. It is the resistance, which mistrusts any new initiatives and fears to have to relinquish habits, even if they are attitudes of imprinted stress.

In addition to that, sometimes there is an inner impatience, which wants to see immediate success: a drastic change or the immediate disappearance of a persistent symptom. However, with this approach many symptoms only resolve towards the end and not at the beginning of the transformational process. When the parasympathicus is strengthened so much that it can act as equivalent partner of the sympathicus and reduce its activities, when they explode without reason, then there is no ground for many stress induced symptoms and they vanish without trace.

3. External Support

Using external support, e.g. with watches, CDs or apps, helps us to find and keep the appropriate breathing frequency. After some time, these tools can be put aside. We acquire a sense of the suitable form of Coherent Breathing for our condition. Then we can go with the free flow by consciously tuning in to the breathing frequency and amplitude as well as regularity in the beginning and include all the components in relaxed meditation in the moment. There is no control needed at this point, no concentration on being aligned with objective parameters. Practicing Coherent Breathing merges with meditation by receding to the background and gives way to the inner experience in the moment. In this we connect the benefits of Coherent Breathing and of mindfulness meditation, which works without regulation.

The body breathes now in the most pleasant way for its needs, and we participate with our awareness. Thus, not only do heart and breathing come to coherence but also body, mind and spirit.

4. Practice as Meditation

The learning process happens also the other way round: In meditation an unconscious form of Coherent Breathing arises by itself after some time of practice. By turning inward, coherence is created on an unconscious level. The value of Coherent Breathing, which arises through relaxation, flows into meditation in this case, deepening and enriching it. As this way of breathing balances the nervous system, it helps the meditating person towards inner calmness and silence. The vagal brake, which is strengthened by breathing exercises, provides the physiological basis for this experience, which allows us to enter the position of the observer or witness: Perceiving inner processes, body symptoms and feelings without identification and without allowing them to dominate us. This is only possible, when we are in the smart-vagus state, or can easily regain it should it be lost. This important ability, the handling of the vagal brake, also helps us in dealing with the problems and challenges of the outer world with more relaxation, without having to enter into the usually unnecessary and counter-productive fight/flight acti-vation of the sympathicus. This is when meditation becomes part of everyday life.

Thus coherence deepens meditation, and meditation furthers coherence. Coherent Breathing starts as structured and regulated practice and easily transitions into meditation by letting go of any structure.

With growing experience in practice, letting go and relaxing on the exhale becomes increasingly easier, simpler and natural. This central component of Coherent Breathing works best without any internal or external demands, in the realm of freedom from expectations, rules and necessities.

5. The Six Bridges

Stephen Elliott has developed the model of "six bridges" out of interest in the "dual control" we have over breathing. It means that we can influence our breathing voluntarily and that it runs auto-matically, when we are not focusing on it, having our awareness elsewhere.

Elliott calls such interfaces in the human body bridges: Parts of the body, which allow conscious interaction between somatic (voluntary) and autonomic neural functions and regulations. These are also parts, in which we can direct the autonomic nervous system in a way that we want to. And they are areas, which are responsible for the inter-active exchange with the world. So it does matter how these areas are set up: When they are tensed, we are closed with shut hatches. When they are relaxed, we are open, we let information in and send it out. So relaxation is connected with a communicative state, and tension with egotism, fear and fight, as can be deduced from polyvagal theory.

Breathing is likely to be the strongest and most influential bridge, as it works permanently, uses big muscular groups in the thorax and cooperates directly and intensely with the circulatory system. Relaxing the bridges has effects on the muscular walls in the arterial trunk and enhances the lymphatic circulation. The exercise of the "six bridges" involves Coherent Breathing throughout the whole process, and conscious and progressive relaxation of the following parts of the body: Face, tongue and throat, hands, diaphragm, perineum (pelvic base) and feet.

The exercise is done in a lying position. Thus gravity works equally on the whole body and blood can flow freely, especially in the brain.

Elliott writes about this exercise: "One of life's challenges it to prevent the buildup of stress and its result, tension, which ultimately manifests as stiffness and discomfort of both body and mind. When practiced daily, The Six Bridges sweeps the body and mind clean of insult and injury, preventing its accumulation, which is really a nervous system matter, i.e. stiffness is a result of 'noise' in the nervous system that results in activation of low threshold muscle motor units throughout the body. Our goal is to minimize this noise and with it, tension. (This is a fundamental objective of yogic practice.) If we fail to do this, the body gradually becomes 'stiff'. As the body becomes stiff, the mind becomes anxious and inflexible."[18]

An acoustic instruction to this exercise can be purchased from the website of the Coherence Institute.

6. Variations of Coherent Breathing

Resistance Breathing (Brown & Gerbarg 2012, p. 32-39)

Like the purring of cats, breathing with slight resistance in the flow of breath activates the parasympathicus and thus creates relaxation. For this breathing method, there are various techniques, e.g.

breathing with pursed or puckered lips, or, when using nasal breathing, with ujjayi breathing, also named ocean breathing:

A slight tension in the throat area produces a scrabbling or purring sound with inhalation as well as with exhalation. This sound can be almost inaudible so that the breath can flow in and out softly. For practice, it is easier to first start with the exhale and later also inhale with resistance. Five minutes should be enough in the beginning for not overstraining the throat area. Besides it is recommended to combine it with the Coherent Breathing rhythm.

Breath in Movement (Brown & Gerbarg 2012, p. 40-43)

The Breath Moving exercise has its roots in Eastern martial arts. It helps to strengthen the concentration on breathing during practice.

- First find a Coherent Breathing rhythm.
- Then move your attention to the face, the neck, the shoulders and hands to relax them.
- Imagine during the next inhalation that you move our breath to the top of your head.
- With exhalation, move your breath to the lowest end of the spine, to the perineum and sitting bones.
- With each inhalation move the breath to the top of your head.
- With each exhalation move the breath to the perineum.
- Breathe in this circuit for ten cycles.

In a further cycle of practice, the breathing circle can be expanded in the body so that it includes head and feet. Combined with resistance breathing, this is a complete program for practice of Coherent Breathing.

Breathing for Relaxing the Jaw

The basic exercise of Holographic Breathing by Martin Jones[19] can easily be combined with Coherent Breathing. In this technique, the lips are closed while the lower jaws sink slightly with the inhale and lift up with the exhale. The tongue is twisted up to the roof of the mouth. With this exercises, tensions in the jaws can be released.

Reduction of Acute Stress by Breathing

When you are under strong stress, relieving the whole body is needed at first, as e.g. by shaking the body connected with vocal expression or by flinging the arms and sighing and moaning the pressure out of the body. So the muscular tensions are loosened through the reinforced and accentuated exhalation. This relaxes the diaphragm and can attribute to breath relaxation.

In the next step, you can work with prolonging the exhalation e.g. in the relation of 2 – 4 – 2, that is breathing in on two counts, breathing out with double length and holding the breath on two counts. Thus the parasympathicus gets the space to become more active.

Finally you can switch to Coherent Breathing by equaling the length for inbreath and outbreath so that the relaxation on the exhale and the Valsalva-wave can by fully applied.

7. Questions Concerning the Practice

Catching Your Breath – The Air is Scarce

When a sudden hunger for air comes up during inhalation, this is due to stress and tension. The fear at work is of not getting enough air. This is similar when seemingly the air is not sufficient for inhalation according to the time necessary for keeping the regular rhythm. It can help to include a small break until the time for exhalation comes and then to breathe out slowly. Newcomers and impatient and stressed people tend to suck in the air too quickly. Such symptoms correct themselves over time of practice. When continuing calmly and consistently, the symptoms will vanish soon.

Five Breaths per Minute are Too Quick

Persons with much experience in meditation or with training in various breathing techniques want to breathe even slower. It is good for meditative breathing practice to breathe very slowly, but it does not improve the heart rate variability essentially. The practice of five breaths per minute can be done with many different activities with slight physical strain and help to find the optimal balance in them (Brown & Gerbarg 2012, p. 25).

Practice with Stuffed Nose

Even when your nose is blocked, we recommend breathing through the nose as much as possible, at least partially. If this is not possible, you can breathe with half closed lips until the nose is free again.

When there is a lasting problem due to allergies or other disorders, it is helpful to breathe with pursed lips, as with a kissing mouth. There is an exercise affecting the meridians to clear the nostrils: Press both fists to the armpits while calmly breathing in and out.

Family Needs

In order to practice, we need a calm and undisturbed place for a short while. This should be communicated to all the other persons in the household so that there are no interruptions. Infants can be included in the practice as they quickly calm down when they are around someone with relaxed breathing (cf. Brown & Gerbarg 2012, p. 23 – 25).

A mother has written that she can "breathe" her small son to sleep who is especially active at bedtime. She takes him to her lap and breathes coherently, till he is asleep. Coherent Breathing is contagious.

Summary:

1. Take your time for exercise: 5 – 10 minutes – more does not harm!

2. Stick to a fixed point in time: favorable: in the morning or in the evening; keeping the same time every day is beneficial for the success.

3. Keep regularity: Daily practice promotes success. Practicing for a short time but daily is more effective than practicing for a longer time with irregular intervals between the times of practice.

8. Biofeedback and Coherent Breathing

In biofeedback, physiological functions are visualized by direct measurement so they can be immediately observed by the experiencing person. The client can try to alter these functions through operant conditioning to a desired direction.[20]. For instance, the device reports the heart frequency via sounds, and when they are too high, the client can try to relax, which is indicated by decelerating sounds. They in turn deepen the relaxation via positive feedback, and as a consequence, the heart frequency is reduced even more.

The advantage of the biofeedback method is obvious: it can visualize various aspects of the vegetative nervous system, so that the client can get an immediate feedback and learn in this way to regulate the processes on the vegetative level. The desired changes can be observed directly and add to the success in training.

When practicing Coherent Breathing, biofeedback immediately provides information about the effects on various physical functions like heartbeat, muscular tension, blood circulation etc. Thus the efficiency of the method becomes evident, which strengthens the motivation to continue with the practice.

The obvious disadvantage lies in the dependency on devices and external measurement. In contrast, training in Coherent Breathing offers the opportunity to regulate inner processes by breathing and monitor the feedback internally. In this way, the inner sense becomes more attuned and gains self-competence. Additionally, Coherent Breathing can be practiced at any time everywhere without any device.

Coherent Breathing as an independent practice is a pure first-person method for health provision and life extension. Biofeedback combines first-person perspectives and third-person perspectives in an interesting way.

Important Points:

Training in Coherent Breathing requires continuity and regularity.

We help our organism to find its way back to its original way of functioning, which enhances our motivation for practicing.

Short Coherent Breathing sessions undertaken on a daily basis are more efficient than longer exercises with longer intervals between them.

Technical aids can improve the success of the exercises and later become secondary.

Under strong stress, we should first shake off the tensions with body-based exercises and calm our breathing down before starting with Coherent Breathing.

Chapter 7 – Other Schools of Breathwork. A Survey

Why should we do other breathing exercises, when we can achieve the best results for our health and inner balance with Coherent Breathing?

Coherent Breathing has one central aim: Training the flexibility of the nervous system. This follows the principle that general flexibility is more important than performance in a particular area. The ability to adequately cope with different challenges and changing environmental conditions is a meta-ability for every specific quality of performance. In addition to that, achievement is always related to situations, for which it is required, and does not have an absolute measurement. A bodybuilder can impress others with his muscles in a fitness studio and as an action hero, but he does not need his muscular equipment for playing with a baby or running a porcelain shop. When he cannot switch from one context to the next and adjust his force to the relevant circumstances, he just causes damage. By applying his abilities appropriately, he will always act correctly.

So Coherent Breathing somehow has the role of being a form of meta-breathing in relation to other methods of breathing. It can be applied always and at any time, between other exercises or daily routine activities. It can be practiced as often as possible to get anchored on the level of reflexes so that we ultimately return to this way of breathing automatically as soon as circumstances permit it.

Other breathing exercises have their benefits and specific effects. They are not overruled or replaced by Coherent Breathing. Rather, they serve the purpose of expanding flexibility and furthering inner growth in a different way. Breathing coherently trains these abilities on the level of the autonomic nervous system, while other breathing exercises have their effects on the strength of the breathing muscles, gas exchange or metabolism, causing quick relaxation or help with expressing feelings.

There are a huge number of breathing exercises, breathing approaches and schools. Breathing offers us a lot of varieties and opportunities to influence our inner systems. Our breathing can be fast or slow, shallow or deep, in any gradation. We can breathe with belly and/or chest, through the nose and/or mouth, we can connect inbreath and outbreath or make pauses in between, just to name the most important varieties. Breath awareness is taught in many schools of meditation, mindfulness trainings, and there are many courses on breath pedagogies and breath therapies. Each of these different breathing methods has its own respective merits and advantages. None of them can provide everything, so we always have to consider our own personal purpose for finding the most appropriate and helpful way of breathing for us.

So we do not have to give up any of the breathing exercises when we start to practice Coherent Breathing. It is helpful in any way to understand the functioning of certain breathing methods as related to Coherent Breathing to be able to find the adequate context of one's own experiences. This is why you get some general orientation in the jungle of approaches, always in relation to Coherent Breathing. For more information in detail see my "Manual of Breath Therapy" ("Handbuch der Atemtherapie", Ehrmann 2004 - parts of the book are also available in English, please contact the author).

1. Schools of Strong and Intense Breathing

When the enforcement of breathing is demanded, which is to breathe more strongly than usual, the production of artificial stress is consciously aimed for. Breathing should be expanded beyond the range of its normal state in speed and volume. When practicing intense breathing, you activate your breathing as if you were undertaking sports, creating a surplus of oxygen and creating a decrease in your carbon dioxide levels without consuming that energy through actual movement, which is through increased combustion.

Schools using enforced breathing as central tool are e.g. holotropic breathing (Grof 1988), Rebirthing breathing (Minett 1994), transformational breathing (Kravitz 2002) and a lot more. They have all developed from psychoanalytical body therapy founded by Wilhelm Reich, Freud's disciple and renegade. Reich himself had used enforced breathing a lot in his work and gave it a crucial position. It is used for resolving mental and physical blocks and for opening the access to unconscious parts of the psyche.

Intensified breathing does not serve the goal of balancing the nervous system as in Coherent Breathing, but to the contrary it works by: breaking through habitual limitations and creating chaotic states in different systems of the body. As a result of this, rigid emotional structures, which have developed as protection against unintegrated traumatizing experiences, dissolve. By widening the volume of breathing, inner boarders are loosened up and become more transparent for original experiences stored and locked in tense and stiff body tissues.

This is why Stanislav Grof used intense and enforced breathing as a replacement for the hallucinogen drug LSD and thus developed holotropic breathwork. This method can generate consciousness-altering and transpersonal experiences as well as memories from early childhood or prenatal life. Leonard Orr, who invented Rebirthing breathing, named this technique in an allusion to birth trauma (Rank 1924), which can be relieved and resolved by breathing connected and strongly.

Increased aliveness, which is frequently experienced with intense breathing, is connected with changes in metabolic processes. Intensifying the breathing metabolism and especially losing CO_2 can trigger unpleasant but also sensual and ecstatic experiences. In the course of a breathing process started with enforcing and accelerating the breathing, first a phase of intense breathing connected with going through strong feelings happens. By resolving impediments the flow of breath becomes softer and gradually a phase of relaxation follows, which can lead deeply into a peaceful and liberated inner space.

In the schools of intensified breathing, the sympathicus gets activated due to enforced breathing. The metabolic acceleration leads to an increased loss of CO_2. On account of this, memories mainly from the procedural storage that were connected with a similar sympathetic activation arise, i.e. previous experiences associated with strong stress symptoms. As we know, stress always causes the acceleration of heartbeat and breathing. After having gone through these intense emotions, the sympathicus calms down and the vagal brake starts to work, which furthers the dominance of the new vagus and its social bonding system. Intense forms of breathwork always include experiences in bringing stress to rest via deep relaxation.

Similar to Yoga asanas, a cyclical principle is put in action: Stretching is followed by resolution and relaxation. The more we stretch, the more we can relax afterwards. Thus we stretch the breathing space and the intensity of metabolism with intensified breathing and can experience ultimately deepened relaxation. In most cases, intense activation of the sympathicus leads to a deeper activation of the parasympathicus.

Such methods of breathing are not recommended for practice in daily life. When they are executed too often, they can cause dysfunctional regulations in the nervous system. These not only enforce chronic stress, from which many people suffer, but also health problems as the heartbeat can lose even more of its variability. So intense breathing methods and breathwork based them should be exercised only within a therapeutically safe setting, except one already has sufficient experience with such methods.

Coherent Breathing can be used for regaining a balanced state of the nervous system after such processes. The inner chaos created by intense breathing can be guided back to a beneficial order structure, where one breathes with regularity and relaxation. So I recommend to all teachers and therapists, who work with methods of intensified breathing, to get acquainted with Coherent Breathing, so they can pass it on to their clients and students for their daily practice.

On the handside, for training in Coherent Breathing it is useful, when physical blocks and fears, which cause them, have already been resolved. The relaxed exhalation as tenet of Coherent Breathing cannot just be acquired by conscious intention, rather the muscular tensions have to be resolved, which are in the way of relaxation. Such muscular blocks have a background in the events of one's life and therapeutic guidance and support is needed for resolving them sustainably.

Some of the breathing schools working with intensified breathing are not only used as methods of self-experience for creating diverting experiences, such as altered states of consciousness. However, in a therapeutic setting this same technique can be used to aid and assist people with severe mental conditions, undergoing a psycho-therapeutic process. Using conscious breathing in psychotherapy is the subject of chapter 11. Furthermore, the Wim Hof-Training is presented as a more recent example of intense breathing methods in chapter 9 in more detail.

2. Dynamic Breathing Meditations

Many spiritual traditions use meditations or rituals with enforced and rhythmical breathing, often connected with archetypical ritualized or monotonous movements, sometimes also with dance. These exercises can happen in a shamanistic context, e.g. derived from tribal rites of North American Indians or from mystical traditions like the Islamic Sufi tradition. There are also intense breathing exercises in the Pranayama school, e.g. fire breathing (Sabatini 2007). Often such exercises aim at creating a state of trance with wholesome and consciousness-expanding effects.

For instance, there is the Ho-Ya Sufi exercise, which consists of breathing in as well as out in two steps and with sounding the syllables Ho-Ya on the two steps of exhaling. When breathing in, the abdomen should be expanded before the chest, and when breathing out, the belly should be contracted before the chest. Thus the volume of the breath is enlarged. Additionally, the breathing rhythm will gradually accelerate: Over a time of ten to twenty minutes, the breathing becomes faster and faster until the absolute maximum in tempo and volume is reached. After that, the breathing calms and slows down and after a short break the next cycle starts. The exercise is closed after two to four cycles with a longer phase of relaxation.

Similar to schools of forced breathing, such forms of active meditation primarily speed up the sympathicus, often close to the border of exhaustion. Then there is sometimes an abrupt shift to the parasympathicus, like the typical "Stop" at the end of the third phase of the dynamic meditation by Osho: Starting with intense breathing, followed by emotional expression and a phase of jumping, which is suddenly interrupted, the dynamic shifts to total freezing. This aims at a similar effect we can notice with sporting efforts: The bigger the physical effort, the deeper and more pleasant the relaxation afterwards. To better understand this phenomenon, see chapter 9.3, p. 114 with the explanation of the concept of hormesis.

Entering intensely into the turbulences of the sympathicus also causes a simplification of thinking, which can withdraw completely in the ensuing phase of silence. Thus a further concern of meditation, the liberation from the activities of the mind and mental cleansing is included.

Such ritualized or meditative forms of breathing result less in working through unresolved emotional experiences; but rather want to initiate a state of trance for the expansion of consciousness. The changes in the gas exchange that occur due to the activation of the sympathicus lead to changes in the blood supply of the brain, which permit novel inner experiences Here we meet ancient traditions and methods, which have been used for ages for tribal purposes, and exercises from mystical schools used for spiritual enhancement for centuries.

In such exercises, blockages in the breathing muscles can be resolved, which are connected to traumatization. This should be considered as part of the whole system of therapeutic support as it needs further integrative work. This is why dynamic breathing meditations should mainly be practiced in groups with experienced leadership so that competent social backup is provided, which can interact directly with the person undertaking the work, and better help with their individual problems.

So far, there is little research on how the environmental conditions of sympathicus activation determine inner processes. It seems that an enforced arousal of the sympathicus during intense breathing exercises done with conscious intention and under safe circumstances, is usually easy to integrate. It can produce quite different inner effects as compared to an activation, which is triggered by aversive fear generating stimuli from outside. In such cases, the inner and outer resources are missing as they prevail in a conscious breathing exercise. Instead, the situation is connected with threat and loss of control.

Traumatizing situations are those, in which we get caught off guard: We are not prepared for the danger and do not have our resources at hand. Consequently, totally different inner processes are at work as opposed to situations, in which the inner arousal happens in a relaxed framework. The maximum mobilization of all available resources and energies, as it is significant for the trauma situation, is not necessary for situations of exercise. When we practice, we are much less in need for help, so even less inner resources are required. Then different inner processes can be activated for the integration of the experience.

It can also be beneficial to build up training stress by intensifying (deepening and/or accelerating) our breathing. This means that the body is put in a state of stress during an exercise, which is not triggered by an inner fear. In the state of training stress the anxiety centers in the brain will not be activated, which normally trigger the stress cascade in the neural and hormonal systems. Rather, the organism gets transferred by conscious intention, into a state, which it usually familiar from situations of strain. Due to the voluntariness at the beginning of the exercise, we keep a sense of control over the situation. Thus we experience physiological stress in connection with cognitive control. By this, the emotional centers in our brain learn to decouple stress as a sensual form of achievement from feelings of fear (cf. chapter 9.5, p. 166).

For a few minutes, we breathe intensely in and out and notice what changes in our experience. E.g. we feel dizzy and sick or energized, alive and motivated. Our body becomes stressed, but it is clear that this is just an exercise, so we do not feel any fear.

After the exercise, we return to balanced breathing and furthermore, have trained our breathing muscles with the exercise. Also, we have directed the attention of our brain on the possibility that intense breathing is not always connected with danger. Thus, we also train the emotional areas of our brain to react more flexibly to situations of strain and the challenges of everyday life.

This is why intense breathing exercises also improve our understanding and inner knowledge about our mechanisms of stress, which helps us to gain competence in handling them. As with to sports or other strenuous leisure activities we enter into a sympathetic state with strengthening effects, from which we can sufficiently regenerate and relax afterwards. We will discuss this topic in more detail in connection with the intense breathing exercises by Wim Hof (chapter 9).

For all those who like intense breathing exercises, Coherent Breathing offers a valuable complementary addition for daily practice and permanent breath awareness. Ritualized breath meditations require certain environmental conditions and consume more time, while we can breathe coherently any time and even for a few minutes. When you have encountered the deep reaching effects of conscious breathing in rituals and meditations, you will quickly understand that slow and regular breathing also has beneficial effects on health and well-being. Meditative experiences, which often get activated in ritualistic exercises with enforced breathing, can also arise in a Coherent Breathing exercise and enrich it.

3. Internal Breathing Meditations

The "classical" silent meditation found in Zen or Vipassana and the manifold schools of mindfulness aim at a state of relaxed calmness as a basic attitude in life. For this, controlling emotions is required, which can happen by perceiving them from a position of a neutral observer. Enticements should be tempered and weakened, which activate the sympathicus without necessity and put us in a state of tension in daily life. We can call the sympathicus an executive servant of fears and desires, which are the roots of human suffering according to Buddhist teaching: When we get activated, because we have to get something we need so desperately or because we have to avoid something in all costs, our nervous system switches to sympathicus activity.

In contrast, silent meditation is considered the royal path to inner relaxation. Many scientific studies confirm that meditation supports the vagal brake. E.g. Porges and his colleagues have found that persons with experience in meditation can better cope with the consequences of traumatization, i.e. they can better cool down the sympathicus.

In addition to that, states, which can be reached by a meditator, resemble the parasympathetic experiences as described above. The devotion of a breastfeeding mother or a loving couple can be experienced in an extended sense in meditation as unlimited love or interconnectedness. This means that we can access a parasympathetic state of specific devotion in meditation, which "misuses" a chemical mechanism developed by evolution for triggering attachment behavior. By renouncing the social purpose, this mechanism can be used for the search for the highest forms of human self-realization. For this speculation I have not yet found any evidence from scientific research.

Be that as it may, our nervous system offers various possibilities; yet to use them also requires a conscious decision. Let us repeatedly start to direct our attention on our breathing and relax the exhale at the same time. By doing this, we immediately approach the peaceful polyvagal state of meditation.

Training breath awareness results in improving and refining inner perception. Thus, breathing can serve as feedback, as a kind of monitor that informs us of our momentary state, and at the same time, that acts as an indicator our current state, bringing us closer to the desired target state.

4. Pedagogical Schools of Breathwork

The pedagogical schools of breathing ("Atemlehre" according to Ilse Middendorf 1990, who taught the "perceptible breath") aim at correcting disorders and inhibitors to the breathing function. The method is re-education: Bad habits of breathing should be replaced by better ones. A large number of exercises are offered, which often combine breathing with vocal expression and movement (cf. Faller 2009). In this context, a detailed explanation is followed by the exercises and, if necessary, the relevant corrections follow. These exercises also improve the inner observation with the main focus of perceiving and changing patterns of breathing and body posture.

Coherent Breathing is also a kind of breath training. For it advocates rules, which have to be followed. The pedagogical goal is to achieve more flexibility in the vegetative nervous system and the strengthening of the parasympathicus. However Coherent Breathing asserts that the natural flow of breath known in breath pedagogics is subject to rather exact regulative demands of the organism and which cannot be achieved by exercises of breath observation and liberation alone.

All exercises, which lead to relaxed exhalation and widened inhalation are beneficial. Yet the Valsalva Wave with its balancing effect on the whole organism, the objective of Coherent Breathing, can only be realized when following the correct parameters that are demanded by the functional needs of the organism.

5. Pranayama

Pranayama is the breathing branch of Yoga. Pranayama means "control of life energy". There are many exercises that are often, but not exclusively done in sitting. One of the goals of pranayama exercises lies in calming and controlling breathing. For this purpose, the disciple counts her breaths on the inhale and the exhale, or extends them by "thinning" the breath, i.e. slowing it down so much that it is hardly noticeable. Also pauses after exhalation or inhalation (*kumbhakas*) are used. Practicing pranayama serves the purpose of cleansing and harmonizing the body and to increase mental clarity (Iyengar 1994).

People with experience in pranayama will easily learn to breathe coherently, which also follows exact rules and subjects the breathing to a relaxed control of inflow and outflow.

6. Summary

The numerous breathing schools, which have developed over millennia and increasingly in the last decades use the various dimensions contained in conscious breathing. All of them have their assets and serve different purposes. They also meet different tastes. They work with emphasizing the sympathicus or parasympathicus or a combination of both.

Practicing Coherent Breathing offers a new dimension of breath experience to people who have practice in intense breathing, because it is done controlled and relaxed at the same time. Emphasizing the sympathicus by enforced breathing is regulated back to a relaxed state respectively brought in balance by the parasympathicus. Thus, the flexibility of the inner systems is improved, which is an important component for gaining stress resistance and resilience.

For people acquainted with softer breathing exercises, Coherent Breathing offers an enlargement of their repertoire for practice and acts as a useful complement. The physiological findings explaining the efficiency of Coherent Breathing can also be transferred to other forms of breath meditation.

Coherent Breathing offers in compact form a breathing method with the most reliable way to create relaxation and to balance the autonomic nervous system. Due to its elaborate theoretical background it can be plausible for many people and by HRV measurement, its physiological efficiency can be objectified and monitored by professionals as well as by amateurs. The pursued goal, optimizing the nervous system, is undertaken in order to create a central key for our well-being and sustainable provision for the prevention of diseases of various kinds. So we can practice any breathing method, when we like it and want to feel its benefits; but we never should forget about Coherent Breathing, it always should be a central and indispensable part of our practice.

The plentitude of possibilities is one of the great gifts of breath in its conscious-unconscious double function. Coherent Breathing can claim a special position among the flowers of this ample garden, as it is able to cause alterations in the regulative circuits of the central exchange and metabolic processes most profoundly. There are other goals we can reach via breathing, and for them we should use the appropriate methods. They all can be combined with Coherent Breathing in fruitful ways.

On the Benefits of Flexibility

More flexibility implies the ability to switch more easily from situation to situation, instead of suffering from unexpected or unpleasant changes occurring in the outer environment: Suddenly traffic stops, I cannot move any more. Instead of getting annoyed I use the time for entering into a state of relaxation. As soon as the jam has dissolved, I switch to the active mode and move on. A task needs longer to be completed than planned, as another person is late with delivering her contribution. In place of indulging in worries about the possible outcomes of the expected delay, I look for other tasks, which wait to be accomplished.

When we are more flexible, we can more easily walk with life – which by itself constantly creates changes, novelties and surprises. This is why the Greek philosopher Heraclitus coined the sentence: "Everything changes and nothing stands still." And Buddha said: "In constant change is the world. Growth and decay are its real nature. Phenomena appear and disappear. Happy are those who observe peacefully." In directing our awareness to our breathing we can realize and experience the changeability and fluidity of life in any moment. With our breathing we can enter, at any moment, into this flow, which we can regulate via our breath awareness.

When you become more flexible, your inner world can better adapt to the outer world, so that a complementary inner change happens together with the outer change. You join into the flow of steady alteration instead of opposing it or distancing from it. For this you need a mobile and adaptive inner area, and on the physiological level you need a flexible nervous system.

A flexible muscle has more possibilities as a tensed and shortened one. When you stretch muscles, they can perform more movements and you increase your degree of freedom. Stretching the breathing space, spatially as well as metaphorically (in the realm of possibilities) gives you more freedom, which can come into effect in different ways: Quantitatively, more "life energy" is available; this is more mitochondrial fuel for the activities of our cells. Qualitatively, you gain more flexibility, which helps you to use a greater degree of energy for creative projects in your life. You can accomplish routine activities quicker as they tend to tire you less, and you find fresh ideas for new projects and the respective resources for their realization easier.

Often, people stick to one method, which had been especially beneficial for them. Some need the "kick" of intense breathing, others look for a calming way of turning inside with soft forms of breathing. Conscious experience of the breath is only valued and practiced in a particular form, while other forms, which could open other aspects of the inner world and influence different regulatory systems of the body, are neglected. To manage different challenges of life in a flexible way, in turn, also requires a flexible way of handling different forms of breathing, specifically in terms of rhythm and volume. The more breathing techniques we are acquainted with, the more we are better equipped to handle the various situations that life has to offer. Each breathing method provides us with tools, which we can use for different situations.

Important Points:

Flexibility is a meta-competence of our organism and our way of living and can be trained by practicing different breathing exercises.

Coherent Breathing can take the place of a meta-breathing method in relationship to other forms of breathing.

Breathing does not only play an important role for blood circulation and the nervous system, but also for the metabolic processes take place in the body as whole that supply oxygen and dispose of carbon dioxide.

For improving our daily breathing it is important to take care of the relationship with the blood circulation and the nervous system as well as gas exchange.

Chapter 8 – Breathing Less: The Findings of Buteyko-Breathing

Dr Konstantin Buteyko, Russian physician and researcher, developed his method of breath reduction in the nineteen-fifties. He had seen a patient suffering from hypertonia breathing stressed and with difficulty. He suddenly realized that he was breathing in the same way as his patient had been, and also suffered from hypertension. Immediately he started to change his habits of breathing, and the symptoms vanished; as soon as he started to breathe as he had before, the symptoms returned. So it was clear for Buteyko that there must be a connection between habits of breathing and blood pressure and that the symptoms can be changed by changing the breathing.

After some time he started to experiment with more and more patients and explored the physiological backgrounds of improvements that he could observe. During his life (he died in 2003) he was able to prove the connection between bad breathing and poor health with thousands of patients. Furthermore, in the case of asthma, allergies and hypertonic disorders, he went on to find a way to ameliorate these diseases without the use of medical drugs.

Buteyko discovered that chronic and stress induced hyper-ventilation is a general cause of disorders, where breathing too rapidly and too deeply causes too much carbon dioxide to be breathed out. However, it took until 1981 for the application of the method to be permitted across the former Soviet Union. The method spread abroad, mainly to Australia and New Zealand and to the US, to the UK and to Ireland from there. As of today, it is recognized by the German Medical Chamber as efficient in treating asthma.

The simple goal of the Buteyko method is to reduce the volume of air to an average amount, which would be three to five litres. Most people breathe too much and thus are hidden hyperventilators; their breathing is too fast and too deep. Buteyko held the opinion that the organism loses too much carbon dioxide by over-breathing, as it comes by exhaling too much.

1. Breathing and the pH-Value of Blood

Carbon dioxide is resolved in the blood as carbon acid and determines the pH-value of the blood. This is important for haemoglobin to pick up and deliver oxygen. The normal range of pH is between 7.36 and 7.44. A lower value indicates blood acidosis, over acidic blood, and a higher value alkalosis.

The norm value for CO_2-partial pressure is between 35 – 45 mmHg. When the pH-value approaches alkalosis (which can happen by exhaling too much carbon dioxide), because the blood contains too little carbon dioxide, the situation can become critical. In this case, the Bohr-effect can be triggered, where haemoglobin sticks to the oxygen atoms in an alkaline environment, so their delivery to the cells is inhibited.

According to the Buteyko school, the most widely spread reason for alkalosis, which is for lack of CO_2 in the blood, lies in breathing too much in frequency and volume, and this is called over-breathing.

When breathing in a normal rhythm with middle depth, about four litres of air get exchanged in one minute (four litres streaming in and four litres out), whereas in more rapid and deep breathing, up to 15 litres can be exchanged. Many asthmatics and people with sleep apnoea breathe in this way, thus generating the amount of air necessary for the body functions. The consequence is over-exhaling CO_2 and with that a reduction of oxygen supply for the body cells in organs, tissues and especially in the brain.

The Restriction of Blood Vessels

At this point it must be taken into account that the reduction of CO_2 can cause a restriction of blood vessels. When breathing exceedingly above the average amount, the arterial vessels can shrink to the half in diameter, which diminishes the capacity for transport to a sixteenth. This reduction forces the heart to increase its pumping activity by 16 times.

Vessel contraction has special effects on the brain, where it is almost solely controlled by the CO_2 blood value. Breathing suboptimally, can reduce the oxygen supply of the brain by 60% (Blackett 2014, p. 91). Or in simpler terms: The more we breathe the less oxygen arrives to the brain (McKeown 2011). Additionally, the contraction occurring in the vessels will cause high blood pressure, as the heart has to provide more pumping action to keep the circulation going.

Lack of oxygen (hypoxia) probably plays a role in the breathing methods of intensified breathing, which triggers specific memory processes due to malnutrition of the brain. They become effective on the psychic and emotional level, which is used in holotropic or transformational breathing. So these approaches act as intrusions in physical processes, which are effective in a limited frame but which are not appropriate for a regular breathing style in daily life.

2. Vicious Circles of Over-Breathing

Over-breathing, the Buteyko term for quick and intense breathing, can trigger even several vicious circles. In fast breathing, too much CO_2 gets exhaled. Consequently, the body demands more oxygen, so breathing has to be accelerated even more. At the same time, the contraction of vessels due to lack of CO_2 results in an increased heartbeat, which requires more oxygen again. Finally, when we additionally breathe through the mouth, the body loses water (42% more as compared to nose breathing). As the blood plasma consists of 92% water, blood becomes thicker when there is a lack of water, the heart has to pump more and cover the necessary supply of oxygen by breathing more.

The organism is supplied with a correction mechanism for the pH-value in the blood, the so-called pH-buffer. The most important buffer for keeping up the acid alkaline balance in the blood is the carbon dioxide bicarbonate buffer. However, with over-breathing more bicarbonate (HCO_3) is excreted through urine (Olsson 2014, p. 207). Together with negative bicarbonate ions, additionally positive ions are discharged with urine, such as the minerals calcium and magnesium. Deficits resulting from these losses can have negative consequences for muscles, brain and energy production.

Nitrogen Oxide

The role of nitrogen oxide (NO) in the human metabolism is also mentioned in more recent publications on the Buteyko method. The production of nitrogen oxide in the sinuses can be one of the reasons, why many people suffering from breathing problems can find relief by consistently practicing nose breathing. For more information see the section on nitrogen oxide in this book (chapter 5.3, p. 76).

Avoiding Over-Breathing

To undertake a self-evaluation of the level of CO_2 in the blood, Buteyko suggests an exercise with the "control pause": After a normal in- and outbreath, the breath is held as long as possible without urge to breathe in. After that, breathing goes on as before. A pause below 20 seconds can indicate a shortage of CO_2, which often results in breathing problems like panting, coughing, breathlessness, clogged nose and sleeping disorders (McKeown 2011). A favourable value is around 40 seconds, which shows that the body has enough supply of oxygen due to sufficient saturation with CO_2.

Olsson (41 – 55) recommends the following exercises for better breathing based on the findings of the Buteyko school:

1. Inhalation and exhalation through the nose alone
2. Breathing with the diaphragm (belly breathing)
3. Slow and relaxed breathing
4. Rhythmical breathing
5. Breathing calmly and with reduced volume.

There are plenty of other exercises in the Buteyko school. Here some examples:

1. Breathe quietly: Breathe in a way that people around you cannot hear it.
2. Deficit breathing: Always breathe with a slight "hunger" for air, somehow like breath fasting: Breathing only when the body really longs for it.

3. Flat breathing: Breathing easily, without effort and as little as possible.

4. Nasal breathing during sleep: To stay with nose breathing during the night sleep, special plasters are used for closing the mouth.

For more detailed information and recommendations for exercises, specially trained practitioners should always be consulted. The method is based on ample experience although why it functions in this way has still not found a satisfactory explanation. This is what the German Buteyko website www.atemweite.de states:

"While the efficiency of the method has been proven explicitly, there are still many open questions in respect to the mechanisms at work, and further studies have to show the crucial factors for the efficiency of the Buteyko method in the end."

4. Buteyko Breathing and Coherent Breathing

Both methods are compatible, as in the case of Coherent Breathing, one cannot "over-breathe". Practicing slow and middle deep breathing as well as nose breathing averts over-breathing. Strengthening the parasympathicus acts as a preventive precaution to stress reactions, which tend to occur less often and calm down quicker as the nervous system gains more inner balance. Moreover, Buteyko breathing as such is relaxing the nervous system by reducing the volume and speed of breathing.

It is interesting that the origin of Buteyko breathing lies in the observation that breath relaxation can reduce high blood pressure. Also Coherent Breathing lowers hypertension, although using a different model of explanation: Hypertension is a result of scarce use of the diaphragm for breathing. When it does not help the blood circulation, as it contracts too little during the inhalation, the pull on the venous blood circulation is too weak so that the venous part of the blood circulation cannot become sufficiently empty. This results in blood congestion according to a term from Chinese medicine. The arterial blood has to be pumped with more pressure away from the heart (Elliott 2016b). For this reason, as already mentioned, Coherent Breathing requires breathing with middle depth. This corresponds to the belly breathing used in the Buteyko method. However, the volume should not be reduced too much in order to attain the goals of Coherent Breathing – shallow breathing as done in some Buteyko exercises will have no impact on the circulatory system.

Buteyko and Coherent Breathing have differing focal points. Coherent Breathing is not specific to asthma therapy as the Buteyko method is. Its primary goal is balancing the vegetative nervous system. It also can help asthma patients towards further relaxation, although they also should try the Buteyko method for their special condition, which influences the carbon dioxide metabolism more effectively and directly, so it can alleviate or eliminate the asthmatic disorder in many cases. Those who want to improve or heal their asthmatic symptoms without the aid of medical drugs (and without exploring the emotional backgrounds of the disease), are well advised to train in Buteyko breathing and additionally, to practice Coherent Breathing.

Important Points:

Enforced and compressed exhalation as well as unnecessary mouth breathing can reduce the carbon dioxide concentration in the blood, which in turn reduces the oxygen supply of the cells.

This is why we should take care to relax the exhale. Unnecessary rapid breathing should be avoided.

Nose breathing should be the rule, and mouth breathing should only be practiced in exceptional cases.

Chapter 9 –Adrenalin-Breathing of Wim Hof

In the preceding section, we discussed the downsides of intense and rapid breathing. Now we shall investigate the arguments to the contrary, finding that intense breathing can also have surprising beneficial effects. The Dutchman Wim Hof has extreme experience with breathing and inner concentration: marathon runs in heat and coldness (barefoot), climbing Kilimanjaro in shorts, without a shirt and in record time, swimming in the polar sea, 80 minutes in the ice where the temperature was only 1 degree etc. We might think, "This is just a nerd who has practiced his entire lifetime in order to gather impressive results and rewards." We can admire such farfetched and astonishing achievements, but what does this have to do with our normal life? The fact is, he has performed some of these extraordinary activities with people, who had no prior training or experience, saves a course comprising of breathing exercises and exposure to cold water as preparation for extreme experiences (Hof & Rosales, 2011).

Obviously, it is possible that such performances could be undertaken by anyone – with the appropriate preparation. The preparatory breathing exercises he engaged with mainly consisted of breathing intensely, taking short breaks and breathing intensely again, so, according to the wording of Buteyko, hyperventilating intentionally and massively depleting the body of CO_2, or, from the perspective of Coherent Breathing, purposefully bringing the nervous system out of balance.

1. Adrenalin-Breathing

What happens when we turn up our breathing, when we start to breathe strongly and intensely, wanting "to build up the energy"? Rapid and deep breathing leads the nervous system into the sympathicus mode. Somehow the parasympathicus does not get any chance to interfere as the exhalation becomes increasingly regulated by the sympathicus as the speed of breathing grows.

In this state, the body's energy reserves get mobilized and our sensitivities are put on hold. We approach the maximum limit of our performance. At the same time adrenalin production is boosted up and this well-known stress hormone is distributed all over the body. This change is clearly measurable after 30 minutes of intense breathing. It brings us into an aroused state, which can be pleasant or unpleasant according to the internal and external situation. People with panic attacks know intense breathing as a fear-laden experience, sportsmen as a virtually ecstatic "kick".

Adrenalin and Immune System

The increased production and release of adrenalin has the effect of making us more tolerant to pain. This is the experience of a football player who only notices at the end of the game, that his foot is aching. In addition, the immune defense gets suppressed. For in the fight/flight mode, which we stimulate with intense breathing, all the available resources are needed on the periphery for coping with the threat. What is not needed immediately for managing the challenge and thus consuming energies, is kept in the background and silenced. This is why we are capable of maximal performance and extra-ordinary activities when we are in this state.

In a scientific experiment, an untrained control group and a group of Wim Hof breathers who had trained for ten days got an injection of dead E. Coli-bacteria. The control group displayed intense reactions in their immune systems (fever, chill). The intense breathers however showed hardly any or definitively weaker symptoms.

The Dutch researchers who conducted the experiment stated that both the acid-alkaline balance and the oxygen content in the blood had gone up and down several times during the cycles of the breathing exercises. They concluded, and this is a new insight, that we are able to influence our immune system by targeted exercises. This opens the chance to fight auto immune diseases with self-control and exercises[21].

Autoimmune disorders are a result of chronic inflammations and lead to severe, often barely treatable diseases. In these cases the human immune system overreacts, so that the body suffers damage from an excess of healing attempts. These reactions become chronic, and this is the autoimmune disease. Yet when we succeed in suppressing the overshooting immune reaction by voluntarily entering an adrenalin state, such suffering can be diminished or healed. This is at least the hope of the scientists who have investigated Wim Hof and his students.

Should further experiments find proof of these results, it would be possible to understand how the nervous system affects the immune system and this would open a door for us to regulate our immune system from a first-person perspective. We could finally find ways to influence autoimmune reactions beneficially by ourselves, via special breathing exercises.

Adrenalin and Cortisol: Better than their Reputation

In this section we will take a closer look at the role of adrenalin. This famous stress hormone is produced in the adrenal medulla assigned by the hypothalamus. After around ten minutes of adrenalin release, cortisol is produced in the adrenal cortex following a signal from the pituitary gland. This hormone protects the body from the detrimental effects of the prolonged over-activation of adrenalin and also is responsible for heightened, longer lasting vigilance, yet on a lower level than adrenalin. Cortisol fills up the energy reserves, which have been depleted by adrenalin, by converting the energies from nutrition to fat and by outsourcing proteins from the muscles and minerals from the bones.

Moreover, cortisol enhances the capability of the immune system as it prepares immune cells, mainly leukocytes, for action and sends them to the location where they are required. Yet these positive attitudes of cortisol have diminishing effects under circumstances of long term or chronic stress.

In normal cases, the release of cortisol is reduced by a feedback system, which turns off the stress reaction. In a balanced life-style, we can overcome and integrate difficult situations in the following healthy way: Tension is followed by relaxation, stress by regeneration.

Cortisol basically serves to aid this process. Lack, as well as excess of cortisol has mental consequences (behavioral disorders, depression, and sleeplessness). Strong and unfavorable changes in the cortisol system happen after traumatization.

The healthy and useful reaction to stress, which is an emergency reaction, can boost up physical performance quickly and calm it down in a timely and controlled way. The adrenalin and the cortisol system closely cooperate for this task. When the stress is too extreme, lasting too long or lacking adequate regeneration afterwards, the adrenalin-cortisol system can come out of balance and cause detrimental consequences.

2. Breathing and Stress Reaction

There is an apparent mutual connection between breathing and stress reaction:

Adrenalin release (e.g. by a fear triggering stimulus) accelerates breathing; and the other way round, accelerating and deepening breathing, as done in certain breathing exercises, causes the release of adrenalin.

So with intense breathing exercises the body activates the stress reaction even if there is no internal or external cause. What we called "stress" in the exercises mentioned above, is named "chemical stress" by researches. The uncommon and erratic changes of the pH-value in the blood in intense breathing exercises, seem to provoke the alarm reaction on the hormonal level although we do not feel stressed or frightened. With some of the people from Wim Hof's group the pH-value rose up to 7.75 (with a usual tolerance range of the pH-value in the blood between 7.36 and 7.44), what was connected to a quite dramatic drop of the CO_2-level.

As is known in science and in the practice of breathwork, a symptom of blood alkalosis, which is a high pH-value, is the "over-excitability of the nervous system". As a consequence of the reduction of Ca_2+ (calcium-ions) in the blood, the vessels contract and the potential for an increased electric conductivity is generated. This phenomenon is often considered as negative as it can be connected with feelings of panic or panic attacks and is experienced as hyper-nervous feeling, mainly when in combination with a loss of control over the circumstances on the outside.

Nonetheless, Wim Hof experiments demonstrated that the nervous system can be influenced consciously by increasing or decreasing the electric conductivity by exercises, that is by voluntary control. Here we see new opportunities for the self-control of one's health.

3. Hormesis and Stress Experiences

Obviously, there is a significant difference: When we consciously come into a stressful experience, by e.g. deepening and accelerating our breathing, the nervous system reacts differently as it realizes that there is no real danger, but just a challenge the organism faces on the conscious and unconscious level.

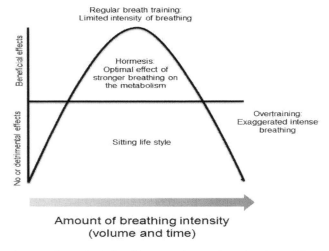

Fig. 12: The principle of hormesis as related to breathing

Although we create a situation of energetic overload, which might trigger memories from previous experiences, we are not as exposed to its frightening sides as we were in the original situation. Here the arousal happens within a stable and safe environment initiated by a conscious decision and thus we have a good foundation for the integration of a previous trauma in the present.

This process can also be understood with the concept of hormesis. It is a principle that was discovered by Paracelsus, and it claims that toxins in small doses can have healing effects. When transferred to intense breathing exercises, it means that stress in partial form or taking place in limited time can improve stress resilience. When we intensify our breathing under controlled and safe conditions, our organism experiences this form of stress as harmless and calculable. With this, it learns to endure stress and regenerate well afterwards.

Oxygen Intake through the Lungs

Due to their elasticity, the alveoli are provided with a large surface for diffusion, used for the gas exchange of oxygen and carbon dioxide. With normal breathing, we possess considerable 70 m^2, which we can even increase up to 100 m^2 by deep breathing. In this way, gas exchange is increased proportionally – there is more intake of oxygen and more release of CO_2.

Wim Hof's breathing techniques lead, according to his statements, to an even larger surface of alveoli. By exercising, more oxygen can be taken in, which leads to more oxygen and less carbon dioxide in the blood. The latter should tend to a minimum, while the increased content in oxygen charges up the mitochondria, the energy producers of the cells. This kind of energy production is called "aerobic dissimilation" or inner breathing.

4. Inner Breathing

Dissimilation is a scientific term for the breakdown of the body's own organic compounds such as carbohydrates, fats and proteins, with the aid of enzymes. This is done in order to generate energy. Dissimilation can happen in the presence as well as in the absence of oxygen. Aerobic dissimilation (with oxygen) is also called inner breathing. Anaerobic dissimilation without oxygen is highly in-efficient. So cells need enough oxygen to be able to produce energy efficiently. This production runs over a multilevel chain, in which a glucose molecule is converted into pyruvate, thus creating two ATP (adenosine triphosphate) molecules.

With enough oxygen present, the process moves on, and one glucose molecule can produce 30 to 32 ATP molecules. ATP is essential for any physical activity, from muscular movements to metabolic processes and the formation of electrical signals in the nervous system. Without oxygen – and adequate nutrition – there is no ATP. With more breathing, there is simply more ATP, while the production of lactic acids is reduced, so that the body stays alkaline. Parallel to this, enforced breathing results in the exhalation of more CO_2, the acid level in the blood moves more into the alkaline range, and this helps to increase aerobic dissimilation.

So Wim Hof thinks that we are able to influence the chemical activities in the body cells with his breathing exercises and that we can turn up the energy production when needed for increasing performance. By doing this, we enlarge the range of abilities our organism is able to perform. It gains more competence, which ultimately increases its robustness and endurance and sustainably safeguards our health.

5. Eustress and Distress

The term eustress was introduced by Hans Seyle, founder of stress theory. Seyle understood eustress as the ability to overcome experiences of stress in a beneficial way. Eustress is in action, when the body has managed and adapted to the difficult situation. Another approach points out that eustress is connected to a positive cognitive reaction on the stressor: The situation is evaluated not as overburdening but as challenging, and this is why there is a positive reaction. In a eustress situation, the persons feel that they are in control of the circumstances and that they will not be helpless in the face of exposure to such situations. A third theory connects eustress with the concept or allostasis. This term signifies the ability to gain stability under varying conditions. With this point of view, eustress is considered as a reaction for increasing the capacity of an organism for the purpose of adaptation. So there is no general agreement on the meaning of eustress. This is due to the fact that there is hardly any research to it, whereas, in contrast and rather interestingly, there is quite a lot of research on its negative counterpart, distress.

We are using the eustress concept despite its terminological vagueness to better understand what happens with intense breathing during training conditions. A characteristic difference between eustress and distress is the level of control over the stress situation. Eustress is characterized by its relationship to the end of strain, and we have a goal we want to reach and the prospect of attaining it. We have decided ourselves to undertake this challenge, and we can leave at any time an whenever we want. So the experience has meaning for us and we have the feeling that we can master the requirements.

Although the physical processes are similar, the inner frame of a eustress experience is diametrically opposed to a trauma experience, in which all these feelings are reversed in the direction of the negative: There is no hope and no meaning in the experience, the pre-valent feeling is of being helpless and at the mercy of circumstances. It seems impossible to overcome or to survive. It is unclear how long the burdening situation will last or if it will find an end at all. The trauma experience contains massive fear, whilst a physiologically similar stress reaction occurring in a practice sequence, can happen without any fear. The neuroendocrine system reacts differently, depending on whether we have control over the situation or not.

Experiments have demonstrated that test subjects who were exposed to stress but had been told before that they would experience a funny scene, reduced their stress hormones faster afterwards. Dopamine and serotonin can be released, and the effect of the stress hormones is weaker, as soon as the experience is over[22]. So positive expectations help in coping with stress.

This means that the experience of stress depends on the context, which determines whether or not it is evaluated as detrimental or beneficial, burdensome or pleasant. We only have to think how we experience running to reach a train, whilst having all the thoughts about what might happen if we missed it – as opposed to a run in the forest for our pleasure, accompanied by the enjoyment of nature and movement. In both cases, the body produces a comparable amount of energy, but obviously totally different hormonal processes are released, which also influence our immediate experience as well as the following phase of regeneration.

So it is not surprising that researchers have found out that when the distress mechanism with its activation of the hypothalamus hypophysis adrenalin axis is used for too long, the growth of cancerous ulcers is promoted, while physical activities connected with sufficient relaxation keep them at bay[23].

Effects Like in Endurance Sport?

Sports medicine and research have shown that training in endurance sports leads to strengthening the parasympathetic system (cf. chapter 12.2, p. 145). It is easy to understand that the heart muscle becomes stronger by sportive training. It gains more volume for pumping so it can transport more blood (up to three times more than in untrained people). The heart frequency in a resting position decreases as the bigger heart is able to transport more blood per beat. As a consequence, the heart minute volume, which is the amount of blood the heart can pump in one minute, can double in people who train. Besides the growth of the heart muscle, the blood volume, the number of red blood cells and the overall haemoglobin rises. This increases the transport capacity for oxygen in the circulatory system, which also increases the endurance capacity.

Consistent physical activity, like parts of regularly performed dynamic breathing exercises, changes several metabolic areas so that resources can be used more economically. This happens with the influence of the parasympathicus, which then can take over more tasks. In balance with the physical strain, inner rest and equanimity is deepened. Many people undergo the efforts associated with under-taking sports activities as they anticipate the overtly pleasant feeling of a relaxed state afterwards.

Wim Hof's exercises, amongst others, aim at training for endurance performance like mountain walking in winter wearing summer clothes. The training includes dynamic breathing exercises, which increase the willingness for experiences of eustress and that tune the organism in this direction. Obviously, the nervous system learns in this way to transform the negative contexts of stress into positive ones, thus turning a distress situation in a eustress experience. During this process, physical performance is decoupled from fear and the organism can reach a new level of inner balance.

6. Dynamic and Coherent Breathing

Again we deal with different goals when comparing these two approaches in breathwork. Also with the Wim Hof practice, we find similarities and differences. Activating the sympathicus in limited phases safeguarded by relaxed environmental conditions, has similar indirect and beneficial consequences for improving parasympathetic performance as endurance sport.

Intense breathing trains the breathing muscles, yet also requires sufficient resting phases to avoid detrimental results from over-training. Those who are familiar with Coherent Breathing can easily find their way back to the balance zone after every form of increased dynamics. So it is recommended to return to Coherent Breathing after each intense breathing exercise. In this way we best take care of sufficient regeneration after any kind of effort by consciously bringing the parasympathicus back into play.

In methods of dynamic breathing, the effect goes top-down: The impulse for a new way of breathing comes from the conscious centers in our brain, which initiate a certain breathing rhythm and motivate the vegetative levels to join in with this vibration. We consciously invest our power and energy in our breathing, approach our habitual limitations and move beyond them. We want to prove to ourselves that we are capable of going further. We force our body into a stress experience, so it produces as much adrenalin as possible. We start to like its pulsation. We want to convince ourselves that we manage to keep up such a high level of charge.

With such practice, we enlarge the space of tolerance of our organism, whether it likes it or not. It has to stretch beyond the limitations of its laziness. It gets trained in this form of flexibility. Somehow as a by-product, it revises its ideas about fear, because it learns in these experiences that intense breathing does not only occur in fearful situations but also under relaxed circumstances without danger or threat. This state is ordered by the higher centers of conscious thinking and supreme control, so either something must be wrong about old programs or they are no longer relevant. Fear conditioning is put into perspective and thus weakened.

Yet we have to consider multiple resistances. Actually practicing requires energy and effort, and it is about overcoming inner impedements. So clearly we possess many different resistances towards overcoming resistances. Consequently we need a lot of motivation and will-power to start the exercises and go all the way through. Usually this is easier to do in a group than it is alone. Only after some time of practice, joy and pleasure come.

On the other hand, we immediately see success when we, for example, master the challenge of encountering with cold water, and are able to take a longer cold shower or dive into icy water. This in turn strengthens our commitment to exercising, and thus we learn that overcoming resistance helps to cultivate a special form of satisfaction. We are no longer subordinate to our resistances but experience actively that we are stronger and more powerful than they are. So we also train our will-power when we perform such exercises.

In Coherent Breathing we somehow work the other way round, bottom-up. We do not expose our body to extreme situations but bring it into a position of rest. By breathing slowly and regularly, we feel an inner relaxation, which is pleasant in itself. The experience of coherence is unspectacular. We do not notice immediately that our heart rate variability has expanded, or that our parasympathicus has gained power. Even with measurements, changes often show as a trend building up over a longer period of time and not simply from one day to the next. In a way, we work subversively and unspectacular. Our nervous system reorganizes itself with every coherent breath, and with every further breath another tiny change happens, until we feel that we have reached a new level. The amendment has worked bottom-up.

An advantage of Coherent Breathing is that we hardly have to face severe resistance. The method is easy to practice, does not require effort, strain or excessive concentration. Persistent commitment is the only attitude, which is required.

A Wim Hof Breathing Exercise

Practicing this technique is completely at your own risk and if you want to do this exercise, make sure that you do not attempt it in water, whilst driving, standing up or without consent of your doctor or medical caregiver if in doubt. Never force yourself and always listen to your body.

1. Get comfortable.

Find a comfortable place to do your breathing exercises where you won't be disturbed. You can sit or lie on your back, but do not do this exercise whilst driving or standing up.

2. Do 30-40 power breaths

Once you are comfortable, you can start to breathe in and out 30 times – not too shallow or deep. Imagine you are blowing up a balloon and your whole body is being saturated with fresh oxygen. This may feel a bit like you were hyperventilating, but you are in control. You may also feel a tingling or lightheaded sensation throughout your whole body, when you do this for the first time. This is perfectly normal.

3. Hold your breath.

After doing 30-40 power breaths, empty your lungs of air and retain the breath for as long as you can without force. During the retention, you can close your eyes and focus on the space between your eyes for relaxation. Just remember to set a stopwatch if you are interested in recording your results. You might want to see how you progress with the breath retentions if you plan to do this regularly over a set period of time.

4. Breathe in for 10 seconds.

After the breath retention, take a deep breath in and hold it for a further 10-15 seconds, before exhaling.

5. Repeat steps 1-4.

Repeat the whole process for another three rounds. Remember to record your times, so you can track your progression.

6. Meditate after 4 rounds of power breathing.

After the power breaths, you can then go into your regular practice of meditation or meditate for five minutes if you are a complete beginner by closing your eyes, bringing your awareness to your breath and focusing on the space between your eyes.

Bonus push-ups:

You can make some push-ups or yoga positions during the breath retention till the reflex for inhalation comes. Notice that you are stronger without air than normal.[24]

Important Points:

Intense breathing exercises can prepare us for extraordinary achievements by mobilizing stress hormones to become, paradoxically, free from stress.

We can become free of fears when we succeed in transforming distress to eustress.

Experiencing stress with dynamic breathing exercises in a limited and controlled frame and in manageable doses expands our possibilities and probably opens new ways for regulating the immune system.

Chapter 10 – Integrative Breathing and Integrative Breath Therapy

Integrative breathing is an encompassing method of breathwork. It works to provide the healing potential of conscious breathing with a broadly diversified offering of approaches, optimally adapted at the specific needs of every client. Integrative breathing is suitable for psychotherapeutic work as well as for deepened self-exploration and for health related improvements of the breathing function. The conscious experience of breathing serves as opener for hidden and suppressed issues so that they can be recognized, worked through and resolved. With professional guidance, the framework for inner experience is secured. By resolving breathing blockages, we also improve our breathing as metabolic function and its interconnection with various health issues. In addition, any experience of conscious breathing helps in refining the inner perception and the exploration of altered states of consciousness.

In integrative breathing, elements of different schools of breathwork are adapted to the specific problems, inner state of development and actual emotional themes of the client. So integrative breath therapy can offer support on three levels: On the physiological plane, with the treatment of special breathing problems, on the emotional plane, with the resolution of emotional issues, and on the spiritual plane, with the desire for inner growth. Actually these areas are interconnected and merge: People who are looking for help with physiological problems discover the psychological roots of their suffering, and persons who want to work on their psyche experience the improvement of their health and physiological well-being.

Integrative breathing as method is in constant development, creating new approaches as different models from traditional breathing schools and other trends in psychotherapy are connected. So it is an open and dynamic model, guided by experience and intuition, consisting less in catalogues of rules to be taught, and more in flexible adaptations of the method to the individual possibilities.

So integrative breath therapists need a broad spectrum of methods and multiple ranges of personal experience with different approaches to breathing. All dimensions connected in the human breathing function are utilized including, letting the breath happen and regulating it consciously, intensifying and deepening it, as well as relaxing and slowing down the breathing. An overall goal of therapy lies in opening the breathing areas, so that breathing can use its full potential (belly, chest and thoracic breathing) without being restricted by muscular tensions.

When working with this method as a therapeutic tool, the familiarity and inner experience with all the developments inherent in breathing is necessary. Only then it can be judged, which way of breathing is the suitable for which moment and for which person for attaining expansion and deepening. How can the breath be used to open the inside, how can what has opened be integrated in a constructive way? How can the core of experience be further explored, and how can what has come to the surface be brought to peace? These are marks of the field, which is put up by integrative breath therapy as soon as client and therapist set out on the joint journey of exploration with the help of breath awareness.

One key aspect is dedicated to exploring the emotional and biographical backgrounds connected to specific tensions and blockages in the breathing spaces. By resolving these tensions, a consistent improvement of the breathing function can be implemented whilst reinforcing psychic and mental health and inner calmness. Additionally, self-competence for dealing with daily challenges better and taking care of oneself with more awareness is improved.

1. What does "Integrative" Mean?

When looking closer, the term "integrative" in relation to breathwork can have four meanings:

1. In conscious breathing, body, soul and spirit come together in an intimate way. The body can be experienced from the inside as unity with the soul.

2. By letting the breath flow (Middendorf 1990), dispersed and shattered parts of the inner world find harmony. In the same way, as the mind combines with the body, also dissociated parts

of the personality can find new connections with the help of the breath as bridge.

3. On a methodological basis, we create the best possible framework for the therapeutic goal of integrating the personality with the breath being at the center of the process and with other additional tools such as therapeutic talk, working with personality traits and with systemic aspects or trauma therapy. Whenever appropriate, the work with the breath is used as part of the treatment for opening the access to the problematic areas of the psyche in a multidimensional way.

4. Integrative breath therapy uses a broad spectrum of methods, which have been developed by the various schools of breathwork. Taking into account the personality structure, the level of inner growth and the physical abilities, the optimal method can be found and developed according to the needs of the therapeutic process. For example, the breathing process can be fueled by emotionalizing music as in holotropic breathwork. But the full attention can also stay solely with the breathing as in rebirthing breathwork. Sometimes interventions from Wilhelm Reich's body therapy are applied to deepen emotional expression, and in other cases conscious breathing is used in conjunction with explorative verbal exchange (Ehrmann 2004, S. 145 f).

The experiences of integration collected in a therapeutic breathing process also result in an improved way of breathing in daily life, which helps the breath student to stay in the presence more consciously and to regain inner balance faster when lost. The achievements of therapy together with relaxing and strengthening the breathing help to include more areas of the physical breathing space into the constantly running breathing mechanism.

2. The Setting of Integrative Breathwork

Generally, integrative breathwork is done in a one-to-one setting. The therapist provides his experience and competence, the client enters into the inner world. Sessions usually happen on a mattress lying down, or exceptionally, in a sitting position (Platteel-Deur 2014). At the beginning, the therapist will explain the method and point out phenomena that might arise during the process. Also issues are spoken about before the process, although some clients prefer to start the session without clear issue, waiting to see what the breathing will bring up.

Every session has its own course and will lead to a harmonious completion: The inner processes calm down and end in a peaceful and relaxed state. Finally the contents and insights from the session are discussed. The therapist can help to bring the experiences into a mental context or find a good inner place for themes still unresolved in the client.

Integrative breathing can also be applied as a form of self-exploration in the group. Usually, the group forms pairs with a sitter and a breather. Then the roles are switched. The facilitating persons take care of the outer circumstances, initiate the processes and complete them. They provide support where needed.

3. Coherent and Integrative Breathing

Coherent Breathing should be recommended as a most important practice for self-support. When clients ask how they can practice in between the sessions, Coherent Breathing is suggested as the method of choice, because clients, who practice consistently in this way, can progress a lot more in the therapeutic sessions as the flexibility and range of breathing has been improved by training. Additionally, the inner sensitivity increases so that inner perceptions are more easily accessible. This improves the doorway to unconsciously stored memories.

4. Integrative Breathing and Mindfulness

Many therapists can confirm that clients, who connect their therapy with mindfulness exercises and meditation, proceed better and faster (Lucas 2012). Practicing Coherent Breathing is both a mindfulness exercise and a meditation in one. It connects with considerable potential health benefits on the physiological side as well as on the mental level.

Yet there is an important distinction between the rules of Coherent Breathing and a basic concept of all methods based on mindfulness. Coherent Breathing requires a controlled procedure (keeping the basic tenets to obtain the goals of this method). It is aimed at achieving a result (balancing the autonomic nervous system and creating coherence between breathing and blood circulation). So it includes action guided by intention.

When practicing mindfulness, any intention and expectation are left aside "on purpose". This approach is about pure perception and experience of what is there, without changing anything about it. Mindful breathing means to breathe in the way the body breathes in this moment without exercising any influence on it. It can be that mindfulness leads to changes in the breathing. But this should not be governed by any intention (Harrer & Weiss, 2016).

Thus the method of mindfulness is based on trusting self-regulation – of the organism and of the psyche –, while Coherent Breathing intends to cause changes in habitual patterns, which have proven to be detrimental. Also when working therapeutically in integrative breath therapy, the therapist often might suggest that the client deepen their breathing or to open certain areas of the body more to the flow of breath. However mindful and accepting attention plays a decisive role: Whatever can be felt internally, should be allowed and accepted free of judgements.

Both perspectives that gently suggest changes and unconditionally accepting what is, are appreciated in integrative breathing. Both are also important for any work in psychotherapy as a combination of first-person perspective and third-person perspective. The mindfulness approach gives instructions to the client (third-person perspective) to direct the attention to the breath (first-person perspective) and to leave aside any impulse for change. In Coherent Breathing, the client is meant to breathe in a certain way (third-person perspective), and can observe inner changes during the practice (first-person perspective).

Important Points:

Integrative breathing is a comprehensive therapeutic method, which uses the breath for bringing suppressed memories to consciousness and uses different approaches offered by the breath for this task.

In integrative breathing, intentionlessness as known from the schools of mindfulness is combined with advice from various methods of breath pedagogics.

Coherent Breathing is a recommended practice for increasing breathing competence and for supporting a conscious way of living for clients of integrative breathwork.

Chapter 11 – Breath Coherence and Psychotherapy

The aim of psychotherapeutic treatment lies in bringing inner conflicts, unconscious urges and other disturbing mechanisms of inner life to consciousness in order to resolves their destructive impulses. "Where id was, there ego shall be", as the famous formula of Sigmund Freud goes.

As with medicine, in psychotherapy it is equally important to direct the view on symptoms and their history as well as on the general inner state. Mental burdens affect the nervous system, and a burdened nervous system affects mood and emotional well-being. When we suffer emotionally, the nervous system gets out of balance. If we want to achieve betterment and healing, we have to regain this balance. Thus, psychotherapy as talking therapy alone without including work with the autonomic nervous system cannot be entirely effective. As humans, we are a unity of body and mind, so psychotherapy always has to work on the somatic and the mental level. Actually, it is impossible to separate them or to consider one independent of the other, as physiology always has an impact on the mind and on our mood, and on the other hand, emotions and mental activities can change our physiology. Thus it is of central importance to take notice of this interlacement in any kind of therapy and to bring psychotherapeutic methods of treatment and interventions in line with it.

1. Mental Problems and Stress

The background of practical every mental disorder can be found in inappropriate and manifest stressful behaviour: depression, panic attacks, posttraumatic stress disorder, compulsive neurosis, attachment disorders etc. These result from situations in our lives that we did not manage to cope with, as they were too intense for us. They increased our inner stress level up to a point, where it solidified to a chronic posture, measureable as elevated sympathetic activation and weak vagal tone. The intimate connection between stress and mental problems has been proven by many studies, thus we can take this as an irrefutable fact.

So stress leads to emotional problems and chronic stress finds its expression in bad moods. As an inseparable ensemble of body and soul our inner sense cannot be in equilibrium when the body is over-strained.

From prenatal psychology we know that human life is sensitive to stress from its very beginning (Chamberlain 2013, Janus 2011). Via the placenta, stress hormones from the mother enter the blood circulation of the child. Toxic influences like alcohol or nicotine can also imprint the stress level of an embryo or foetus. The earlier such burdens occur the more difficult it is to integrate them. This is why many babies are born with a chronic stress pattern (Renggli 2013, Janov 2011). Over the course of the child's life, they can develop into mental disorders and diseases.

Here follows an example from scientific research: Even at the age of fifty, persons who were subjected to strong stress in early childhood had a diminished regulatory function of the parasympathicus, as one study has proven (Wittling & Wittling 2012, p. 249).

2. The Importance of HRV for Psychotherapy

The significance of heart rate variability as measurable indicator for health and resilience is more and more recognized in medicine. Equally important is this aspect for psychotherapy. Therapists who are aware of this phenomenon can value the importance of autonomic physical processes for the functioning of the psyche and include this source of information in therapy. Mental and emotional states are expressions of the current state of the autonomic nervous system, which can be measured and represented by the figures from heart rate variability.

By understanding heart rate variability, psychotherapists are encouraged to,

- Pay more attention to autonomic physical processes,
- Help to build up trust in the organic wisdom,
- Interpret symptoms as expression of failed inner cooperation and distorted inner communication,

- Support in building up improved adaptability (higher variety in behavior, thinking and experiencing) and flexibility,
- Recommend physical methods for improving HRV like endurance sport and breathing and relaxing exercises.

A therapist with experience in Coherent Breathing can give their clients a tool, with which they can effectively increase their heart rate variability, find more inner rest and improved health.

When working with improvements in physical awareness, we create a link to our origins on a very deep level: We all started our lives as an organic process seeking and constructing its autonomic regulation. This is where the foundation of the personality is laid down, and here the attention to undertake inner work should be present. Only when this part cooperates, can inner healing be a sustainable success.

3. Types of Attachment

Let us take the example of attachment research. It distinguishes between secure and insecure attachment between mother and baby in early childhood. When the child has a secure attachment pattern, it can cope with the stress that is created when it is left alone by the mother for a short period of time. It can express its pains and disappointment when the mother returns, and allows the mother to pacify it. In an insecure attachment pattern, stress is also created but the burdening situation cannot be calmed so easily. There are three types of insecure attachment.

In one case (insecure-avoidant attachment), the child acts as if everything were fine, and it hardly takes notice when the mother returns. Yet its inner stress level is very high. The child has already learned that there is no use in protesting. With the help of unconscious mechanisms, it can suppress the feeling of disturbance. The prize lies in perpetuating a stress pattern (Siegel 2009).

In the other case (insecure-clinging attachment) the child is fully active to prevent the mother from leaving. It reacts with strong emotion to the separation. When the mother comes back, it shows a mixture of clinging and anger. It is hard for the mother to pacify or distract it.

In the third case (disorganized attachment) the child is so insecure and stressed that it does not know how to behave. It appears distant, confused, fearful and tensed when the mother offers contact after a short separation.

Such instable attachment patterns, which were explored with infants at around the age of one, can have their roots in prenatal experiences, e.g. when pregnancy was unwanted (Hidas & Raffai 2006). In most cases, they prevail and also coin the adult attachment behaviour as well as the attachment to the persons's own children later in life. With insecure attachment, the associated stress patterns become chronic and get reinforced by all similar experiences of relationships over the course of life.

Insecurity from insufficient attachment situations manifests as deregulated nervous system. The attachment system is para-sympathetically modulated and closely connected with the anxiety system (Hüther & Sachsse 2007). For a basic regeneration of the shattered autonomic processes, practicing Coherent Breathing can be of great benefit. With conscious breathing, persons with attachment insecurities can start to build up a safe relationship with their bodies, as first step for healing their attachment pattern.

4. Example Trauma Therapy

The term trauma has gained more and more significance in psychotherapy. It has a wide definition: Every event, which trespasses the ability of an individual to cope with it, is a psychological trauma. Traumas cause enormous stress and can create long-lasting distur-bances to the self-regulation of the autonomic nervous system. These become obvious in the symptoms of post-traumatic stress disorder: flashbacks, nightmares, heightened sensitivity, sleep disorders, increased jumpiness and hyper-vigilance, concentration problems and emotional irritability. Also social withdrawal, depression and psychosomatic diseases can occur (Ogden et al., 2006).

Bessel van der Kolk, founder and director of the trauma center in Brookline, Massachusetts considers four steps important for trauma healing: Trauma patients "have to find a way to reown body and mind (…) In order to able to do this, most people have to (1) find an opportunity to calm down and to re-focus; (2) they have to learn to keep up regained calmness also with images, thoughts, noises and physical sensations that remind them of the past; (3) they have to open up to the opportunity to be totally present in the moment and to engage with other people around them; and (4) they do not have to keep secrets to themselves any more, also not about how they managed in the past to safeguard their survival." (Van der Kolk 2015, p. 243f)

Coherent Breathing qualifies specifically for the first two steps of trauma healing. The necessary inner pacification consists in reinforcing or even re-installing the "vagal brake". For this, the para-sympathicus-system needs to be backed up, which is one of the main effects of Coherent Breathing. With this help, traumatized persons can be more present in the actual situation and take up social relationships as well as openly talk about their history. Conscious breathing always brings the mind into the presence and anchors the present awareness in the body. Relaxation through conscious exhalation activates the ventral vagus and thus our vagal social competences.

It is also possible to maintain inner presence even when intense and unpleasant feelings and body sensations arise during the thera-peutic process. A therapist, who has learned to direct the client's awareness back to their breathing, will successfully guide them to completion through the process of trauma healing, especially when the client is already experienced in Coherent Breathing.

So Coherent Breathing fulfills all criteria for being included in the standard toolbox for trauma treatment, in clinics as well as in private psychotherapeutic practices – and, as already mentioned, in refugee and reception camps in areas of catastrophe.

5. Example Depression

Many studies could prove that patients with depression have a reduced HRV as well as increased heart frequency. This constellation is typical for chronic stress[25]. So it seems that depressions are connected with disorders of the heart function. This also points towards the fact that depressive persons suffer from a significantly higher morbidity risk from heart circulation diseases as compared to normal persons. Furthermore, people with heart diseases have a higher risk of dying with an additional depressive disorder.

Besides treatment with drugs and psychotherapy, which should be recommended by a responsible-minded physician, simple exercises from Coherent Breathing offer an effective help. As already mentioned above, such exercises can be practiced at any time without effort. People with light or medium strength depressive illnesses need to commit to consistent practice with regularity. Then not only will their mood lighten up and their sleep will improve, but also their self-esteem will grow, as they notice that they can take charge of their healing, even if just a little bit. I often observed that clients with depression achieved significant and long-lasting improvement of their condition just after a few weeks, when they practiced with discipline and commitment.

It is possible to assume that one explanation for this might be the influence of the vagus on the brain, as some studies have suggested (Brown & Gerbarg 2005). The vagal pathways to the brain influence brain centers which are preoccupied with controlling emotions and moods: *Locus coeruleus*, orbitofrontal cortex, insula, hippocampus and amygdala; in addition to that, slow and deep breathing stimulates the neuronal pathways underneath the diaphragm and at the same time activates the above mentioned pathways to the brain, which might have an influence on symptoms of depression.

Furthermore, the already mentioned "youth hormone" DHEA might play a role as a mood elevator. Research supposes that DHEA increases the serotonin concentration in certain areas of the brain and thus acts like an anti-depressant. There is strong evidence that training in heart rate variability considerably increases the DHEA level. This might also be true for Coherent Breathing.

Newer studies indicate that a combination of physical exercises, mainly endurance sports and meditative practices, among which we can include Coherent Breathing, are especially successful in the treatment of depressive persons[26]. What has been well-known to therapists for a long time is thus proven scientifically: Many persons suffering from depression can get over their mood swings with discipline and self-motivation. Constant physical movement and breathing exercises can cause a surprisingly fast improvement in well-being.

However with very severe depressions, the problem of motivation can get in the way of this effective form of self-support: The depressive person needs to overcome his drive paralysis to start with breathing exercises, when the success can only be felt after some time.

6. Psychotherapy: Guidance and Self-Competence

In psychotherapy, the specific issues that burden people, are worked on: Issues in relationship, inner disturbances, specific or unspecific fears etc. In many therapeutic approaches, e.g. in depth psychology, the roots of problems that need to be discovered lie in early childhood or in prenatal experiences. By going through the emotions from that time, the problems should resolve. In other approaches, e.g. in behavioral therapy, strategies are developed, which allow to cope with problems differently in the present context.

Therapy takes place in groups or in single sessions. Anything a client can do for himself to make the therapy more efficient is a valuable and indispensable complement to any therapeutic work. Thus the client learns to help himself in part. For this purpose, Coherent Breathing as form of daily practice and as ongoing training in awareness is very appropriate.

Clients, who learn to relax their breathing and to build up and stabilize breath-heart coherence, lower their basic stress and gain more quality in life simple by doing this. They can access the roots of their issues simpler and faster, or instead, can develop and implement alternatives for action with greater ease. They also realize that they can actively participate in their healing, in daily life as well as in therapy. Moreover, they develop a reliable competence in self-perception in the moment, which is of support for any kind of therapeutic work and increases one's own quality of life.

It is also part of the responsibility of the therapist to point the clients towards this aspect of self-therapy and to suggest and offer helpful and effective methods. Thus the client's autonomy is strengthened and the dependency from the therapist as a person and from the therapeutic process is relativized.

7. A New Paradigm for Mental Health

The health paradigm I have proposed in chapter 1.2 is equally important for psychotherapy. Therapy is not just the matter of the therapist as an expert guiding the healing process. Rather, therapy is the product of cooperation between therapist and client.

Clients become co-creators in therapy, when they learn to better perceive and regulate their inner world. Becoming aware is initially becoming aware in and with the body. Breath provides the bridge for that: Breathing, we become aware of how we feel. Via our breathing, our inner state is reflected. Additionally, we can also regulate the inner state by influencing our breathing. What has lost its balance internally, can find its way back to coherence.

Mental disorders are often signified by extremes. A depressive person complains about having too little drive, a maniac suffers from too much activation. Yet the basis for these two and many other illnesses lie in the same distortion of the vegetative nervous system: A dominating sympathicus and a weakened parasympathicus. This imbalance is characterized by latent fears, which lead to blocking motivation for action in the case of a depressive person and urge for ongoing activity in the other case.

Thus the differing methods of psychotherapy basically strive just for the same: Re-establishing a healthy equilibrium between sympathicus and parasympathicus. To achieve this goal, in most cases the over-activation of the sympathicus has to be reduced, while the parasympathicus gets reinforced.

By practicing Coherent Breathing, these two approaches can be combined – two birds with one stone. Calmed breathing lessens the power of the sympathicus and empowers the parasympathicus. Due to the relaxed body posture during exercise, the sympathicus only needs to be present slightly, while the parasympathicus can play a stronger role. By practicing Coherent Breathing, the organism gets more and more used to the reversal of the relation between sympathicus and parasympathicus, which has been prevalent up to the point of engaging in the work of Coherent Breathing.

Whatever the client does, whatever method is used in therapy to balance the nervous system internally: The progress of therapy is supported by practicing Coherent Breathing, which accelerates the healing process. On the other hand, people with severe traumatization can only open up to verbal therapy with a re-regulated vegetative nervous system. Such clients first have to find peace on a deep level, which cannot be accessed by verbal language, but takes place somewhere in their 'guts' or on a more instinctual level. From here, they can develop the ability to regain this relaxation again and again. Often it is the case that we can only achieve wholesome changes in therapeutic talk, when the strategies of coping with stress have been established and stabilized on the vegetative level. The fundaments of trust are based on this, and it is upon this foundation of trust that all psychotherapeutic work depends.

Case Example:

F. comes to therapy as she has noticed that she easily becomes stressed when she encounters challenging situations at her work. Irrational fears come up. By no means can she allow any mistake, as there may be unforeseeable consequences: People might come to harm on account of her actions, and this is something that she would never forgive herself for.

In the therapeutic work, her birth process becomes the central theme. Her mother suffered from gestosis, a dangerous metabolic disease at the time of her birth. Together with working on the fears connected with this experience, I suggest that she take some time everyday to observe and relax her breathing in order to establish a regular and calm breathing rhythm. Over time she can include the exercises in her daily activities, and eventually, she reports that she experiences the exercises as very pleasant. In only five sessions, she feels such a significant improvement to her symptoms that she finishes her therapy.

Case Example:

R. looks for therapeutic support as he notices similar patterns cropping up in his new relationship as those he experienced with his ex-wife. Not long divorced, he notices now that he becomes extremely angry as soon as he gets the feeling of being rejected by her. He knows this feeling well from his previous marriage and is shocked to notice that the reaction is the same with the new partner. Furthermore, he understands even less, why he so easily reacts aggressively to his children.

The therapeutic work leads back to the attachment history in his childhood. At the age of one, he came to an aunt and was only occasionally visited by his parents. At six, his mother suddenly arrived and took him back from the aunt to live with her and R.'s father. R. thus left the countryside and from the safe place with his aunt and suddenly found himself in a cold and loveless parental flat in the city. He could not conform to the wishes of his parents and was constantly exposed to their anger and rejection. In the therapeutic process, an even deeper root of his fear of rejection was revealed: The experience of not being wanted in early gestation.

It becomes clear who R. is really angry with. When this root trauma is brought out into the open, R. can better understand his own severe history and consequently the feelings of rejection become weaker. As he works with breathing and awareness exercises for calming his nervous system between the sessions, deeper feelings arise after a month of therapeutic work: R. reports that he feels sadness arising repeatedly during the day, which distracts him from his obligations in work, but which also connects him deeper with himself.

So there is sadness behind the anger, the emotional pain about the ruptures of his early relationships has come up. The path to healing can go on in good form. Practicing consistently has added a good deal to this. The feeling of sadness is closer to the parasympathetic nervous system than aggression, which represents an aspect of the stress mechanism and is moderated by the sympathicus. By balancing the nervous system, R. obviously is able to activate the vagal brake better, which reduces the fight-flight mechanism. Thus the body-mind system can allow the rise of deeply stored feelings of pain and sadness.

8. Interplay of Therapy and Breathing Exercises

Whenever clients are ready, the interplay of therapy and breathing exercises works optimally. Daily exercises help to re-regulate mis-managements in the autonomic nervous system, while therapy works on making basic changes to what has caused the original failure. Thus the client notices progress in therapeutic work more clearly as obvious changes appear in her daily life. At the same time, she develops her own competence to better rebalance disturbances and deregulations.

By reinforcing inner perception, she has a diagnostic tool at her hand, which can give her accurate information about her relevant state of activation and can point out to her when to apply changes: in her thoughts or in her actions. And she has this tool with her at any time to influence and regulate her state by herself. Breathing practice includes the additional benefit of directing the attention from the out-side to the inside and thus empowers and sharpens the inner senses.

9. Coherent Breathing during Therapy

Awareness of the breathing is a central part of my therapeutic work, regardless of whether I primarily work on the level of talking or include body and breathing explicitly. It proves constantly beneficial to ask clients to be aware of their breathing when an issue is to be explored with the help of the inner sense. The task of psychotherapy is sometimes described as an integration of dismembered parts of the soul by bringing them to consciousness. Such issues can only be found internally, less via thinking and more via emotional experience in the body (Roth & Strüber 2014), and this is especially true for early themes from a time before the emergence of verbal language. These issues are stored in the implicit or procedural memory and become conscious as physical sensations. For working with them, we need to connect with our inner senses, bypassing the verbal and working directly via body and breath.

The internal channel only opens when we have reached a certain level of relaxation. Tension is characterized by fixating the attention on stimuli from outside – we are in a posture of readiness for flight or fight, whether we are aware of it or not. In any case we direct our senses towards a possible threat. We are hardly aware at all of what is going on inside. This reaction only should provide the necessary energies that we can defend ourselves efficiently or run away in time.

Thus in therapy the ability to calm down, at least a little, is needed. So we need the ability to guide the nervous system out of the dominance of the sympathicus. Without the cooperation of the smart-vagus system, therapeutic work is hardly possible. Many therapists start their sessions by giving the client a little time to come to himself and to feel himself, often by suggesting to direct the attention to the breathing and to relax with that. Then issues arise from the inside, which become the focus of work.

The setting and the persona of the therapist should add to build up trust in the client. Otherwise it will not be possible to build up therapeutic contact or an atmosphere in which the client can open up. Additionally, relaxing the breathing helps to assist the client to come back to that beneficial atmosphere, when it has been lost in a previous phase of the work. When the client has collected experience with conscious breathing, this instrument can be used quickly and simply at any point of the therapeutic process, when the inner contact has weakened.

10. Coherent Breathing for the Therapist

As mentioned above, a trusting atmosphere is an indispensable basis for any therapy. Only a relaxed therapist can radiate confidence and a feeling of safety. This basic attitude acts as invitation for the client to open up and also share delicate and unpleasant subjects.

Clients are usually very sensitive to disturbances of the therapeutic relationship, be it inattention, application of pressure, judgment, critique etc. from the therapist. They quickly withdraw internally, which interrupts the therapeutic process. This retraction usually happens unconsciously; some clients do not even notice that their trust is reduced or totally gone, and they are even less aware about why this has happened. This is not their task, rather the therapist needs the sensitivity to notice when the contact has been weakened or disrupted. Then the issue can be addressed, and when this happens with a respectful attitude, the disturbance can be cleared easily.

Impartial therapeutic presence required for such critical phases in therapy can only be maintained when the therapist is in the same way connected with the client as she is with herself. The best and simplest way to stay in contact with oneself is through breath awareness: When the exhalation feels relaxed, the breaths are middle deep and regular, then the therapist is in a smart-vagus state, a condition granting the necessary degree of trust and safety to the client.

From research and reports about the mirror neurons (Bauer 2005) we know that empathy, the ability to feel with other persons, is only possible when we are relaxed. Under stress, we cannot enter into the world of others. Therefore, the focus of the therapist should always monitor their own breathing, which shows them, whether they are in a state of relaxation, which is in a state of empathy. Yet if the therapist's own issues are triggered as counter-transference, which interferes with the attention reserved for the client, it is again breath awareness, which can lead the therapist out of a momentary self-entanglement. A few coherent breaths will quickly resolve the inner arousal or tension.

A therapist trained in Coherent Breathing has an effective tool at hand for returning to empathic rapport when it is lost: Remembering one's own breathing, trained by consistent practice will suffice to bringing therapeutic presence fully into effect.

Even when a client has lost the fundament of trust with the therapist in a critical phase of the process, this will not last for long, if the therapist reacts openly and accepting. When she stays in her trust or regains it quickly, she soon will succeed in re-establishing the bridge to the client.

Walk your talk: As therapists, we should only suggest exercises to our clients we have tried ourselves. Every method has its peculiarities, which we only get to know by undertaking sufficient training. Besides, we should only recommend a regular exercise, when we ourselves have stuck to a similar practice and have collected various experiences from that.

When you have given Coherent Breathing a try for yourself and found your personal form of exercise, you will soon be fond of it and hardly want to miss it, for it is a simple method that sustainably improves your own quality of life and your competence in work.

Important Points:

Problems that people bring to psychotherapy sessions are in some way always connected to stress, which is an imbalance in the autonomic nervous system.

With any psychotherapeutic method we work with, Coherent Breathing can be used as helpful tool, both for the client and for the therapist.

Experienced in breath relaxation, clients can quickly and more easily access their internal world and thus work with more deeply rooted issues.

Therapists with experience in breathing use their breath awareness to feel when they are distracted and to regain their openness and presence.

Relaxed breathing helps the therapist to keep up the empathic state.

Chapter 12 – Areas of Application

There are many fields in the wide space of human activities, in which Coherent Breathing can be helpful and beneficial. In this section, three areas are picked out from all the possibilities and are discussed in more detail, and the reader's imagination will hopefully create a lot more ideas for using this method fruitfully in service of promoting health and well-being.

1. Coaching

In the area of coaching work, a central issue arising for companies is stress, which appears to rule in many organizations and which seems constantly growing under the circumstances of modern economy.

Coaching clients are less likely to seek help with deeper personal problems, as they do not want to be considered unstable by their peers and colleagues. Often they see themselves as well-functioning members of the company they are working for. When they make use of coaching, it often has to do with feelings of exhaustion, demotivation or overload.

By describing their symptoms, they state that their autonomic nervous system is out of balance. The sympathicus system dominates while the parasympathicus cannot dampen its opponent. Of course there are circumstances in the outer environment that need to be changed for the mood to lighten up – changes around the work and its organization, times for recreation, alteration in habits, conflict mediation etc.

However, the basic key to recovery does not lie in avoiding or alleviating various stressors, but rather, in better organizing daily routine operations. This key is situated internally, connected with deeply rooted patterns, which in today's work environment are often linked with survival patterns. These have influenced the vegetative nervous system over decades by establishing autonomic mechanisms, which become so deeply ingrained that the person believes that it is normal to feel stressed, even if it makes him exhausted and sick.

So, the basic internal organization has to be taken into account for improving the quality of living, as even if we leave a strenuous working place and accept a new job, we take the pattern of over-loading ourselves and overlooking the first signs of overextension and self-exploitation, with us. Should we decide to take a few months off, this does not change the tendency of self-denial that we have carried with us for a long time. We can change such habits only from the inside, e.g. by introducing new habits, which serve our equilibrium and stress resistance. For this, practicing Coherent Breathing is an excellent method.

Furthermore, problems with communication, which can become a topic in coaching, are connected with stress. When someone is in a state of tension they are ruled by a dominant sympathicus, cannot listen well and will easily get angry, as is clear from the insights of polyvagal theory explained in chapter 2. So it is important to be able to relax well for business talks to be effective. And when you are relaxed, your colleagues and customers will experience you as friend-ly, polite and likeable.

With Coherent Breathing, we can offer a simple tool to every coaching client, which he can use to practice and improve his relaxa-tion. Awareness on breathing will also help him to better cope with stressful situations and the manifold challenges in business.

Moreover, Coherent Breathing is helpful for times of regeneration, specifically for improving the parasympathicus. Combined with other ways of relaxation or sportive activities, conscious breathing in a calm and steady rhythm can be of beneficial service for people who suffer from the strain of working life in an increasingly demanding business world, so they can find inner balance more easily.

The solid scientific foundation of Coherent Breathing breaks down the barriers that more skeptical customers of coaching might have. They can be sure that this is not an esoteric fashion trend, which sometimes works for dubious reasons and then does not. Rather, it is a careful adjustment of physiological systems, something we may need at any moment of our lives.

With conscious breathing, we cannot solve all the problems we may have with our job or reduce the demands that have to be met.

However, we can learn to take care of our inner balance even though the expectations of working life grow and grow. When we realize how important but also how sensitive the equilibrium of our nervous system is and what the consequences of permanently losing it are, we will do better in motivating ourselves to take the time for conscious regeneration after each phase of strain or emotionally burdensome situations. And re-establishing the contact with ourselves in more depth will motivate us to reflect on our rhythms in life so that we plan enough leisure time, in which we can regain our inner balance. This is where Coherent Breathing is an invaluable tool as it can be practiced at any moment, as soon as we remind ourselves to take a break and care consciously for our relaxation.

Breathing coherently for a few minutes, can work small miracles. Intense unpleasant feelings resolve, nagging thoughts and worries calm down, new perspectives in seemingly dead-end constellations appear seemingly out of nowhere. Practicing breathing with commitment and endurance can turn us into new people, who attract admiration from others for their equanimity and light-heartedness. Furthermore, breathing training is a simple practice and an excellent opportunity for stress prophylaxis and resilience enhancement against overload, burn-out and other typical manager's diseases. Moreover, it is an essential contribution to long term strengthening and stabilization of our health.

HRV-biofeedback has been used successfully in organizational health promotion and prevention of disease. Employees can improve their abilities in relaxation and concentration individually and in a short time. The autonomic balance measured by HRV increases and subjective individual stress perception sinks[27]. Combined with the individual practice in Coherent Breathing, changes for the better are inevitable.

"Physiological coherence is the platform on which health, happiness, smart thinking, improved performance, better relationships and greater influence is built. Learning to be aware of our energy reserves and how to breath properly to protect them, harness them und recuperate our energy is therefore the critical

first step to complete coherence and Enlightened Leadership."
(Watkins 2014, p. 75)

2. Coherent Breathing in Sports

"Sufficient physical activity especially in the form of endurance
sport is, as proven by all relevant studies, the most important
single factor for maintaining and improving health, exercise
capacity and fitness as well as for decreasing age related risks for
dementia and other age diseases." (Wittling & Wittling 2012, p.
311)

A study in Germany showed that 20 – 25% of all health related
costs are caused by a shortage of exercise, and 14% of deaths are
connected with it (ibd.). Günter Enzi thinks that endurance sport is
the most important way to balance and to the center of the body for
the post-modern office person (personal communication).

Regular sportive activities are obviously indispensable, when we
are interested in our health. Supporting the parasympathicus seems
to play a special role like it happens in endurance sports:

"Through regular sportive activities – especially endurance
training – the parasympathicus starts to dominate by switching to
regeneration, general metabolic economization and emotional
damping in the sense of increased 'inner calmness' and evenness.
In parallel, the organs stimulated by the 'achievement nerve'
sympathicus – among others the hormonal system with its glands
producing performance hormones (adrenalin, noradrenalin etc.)
and functional adaptations (economization of all metabolic procedures) – increase their capacities for achievement in the sense of
a heightened general psycho-physiological performative power."
(Weineck 2004, p. 59, transl. by the author)

The aim of endurance is to develop more endurance. To achieve
this effect, strenuous activity should become the norm. When we
exercise by way of highly active sports like short distance running, it
is only the sympathicus governing the neuronal systems that is at
work. This leads to a high consumption of energy mainly derived from

inefficient anaerobic combustion. Endurance training however furthers the parasympathicus, which directs the organism, despite the moderate yet constant strain, towards calmness and regeneration. This is why performance can be kept up for longer periods of time.

Studies have even proven the positive influence of sportive activities on the epigenetic mechanism in a way to reduce the ageing process and inhibit the outbreak of cancer, especially when the exercises are combined with a form of meditative practice[28].

Measuring heart rate variability has a prominent place in high-performance sport and increasingly in popular sport. More and more sportive persons use the technological opportunities of measuring the heart frequency to monitor their HRV and use it for planning their training. With this they realize the significance of phases of re-generation and can avoid the symptoms of over-training.

Yet the significance of regulating the breathing for empowering the parasympathicus is still not well known. Coherent Breathing can be of good use for improving regeneration after sportive performance. Also during the activity, breath awareness can be supportive, when allowing a maximum of relaxation by keeping the breaths as long as possible without strain. When we succeed in maintaining nose breathing during running or cycling, we promote our health even more. For the nitrogen production via nasal breathing is beneficial for our lungs and thus adds to our capacity for achievement and for regeneration.

3. Coherent Breathing with Children

Coherent Breathing does not have an age limit. Children can start from early on to tune in to conscious and regulated breathing. The first experience should be via their consciously breathing parents or other adults. The resonant space created by the adults includes the child, whether it breathes with the rhythm or not. Breathing is highly infective for joining in to the same rhythm. It is helpful to first tune in to the rhythm of the child and then slowly decelerate it, if the child is breathing too fast and hectic. In this way, the child's breathing function can also be brought to more regularity and evenness. As children are very open to nonverbal resonance, shared breathing with careful modulation offers a good opportunity to calm down babies and infants.

We have to consider in general, that children have a higher resonance frequency than adults in most cases. So they breathe quicker simple because of the smaller seize of their lungs. When we get to know the breathing rhythm of a child, we will soon realize when it is in a good rhythm and when it has lost its inner coherence.

There are many child-friendly and joyful exercises with breathing and there are no limitations to fantasy and creativity. E.g. imagine blowing up of balloons or forming soap bubbles, opening and closing the fingers while breathing like a flower, using the lip brake (blowing up the cheeks and then slowly exhaling). There are also many yogic breathing exercises available for children, and they often like to do them when instructed well by adults.

We are living in times of shockingly high consumption of psycho-tropic drugs by children. The increase rates in this area are alarmingly high[29]. As many children suffer from anxieties and "inappropriate social behavior", we as adults have the responsibility to look for alternatives so that they can start to support themselves to manage their inner states without depending on chemical substances with problematic side-effects.

Coherent Breathing is a method every child can learn and practice. It can help to better cope with the challenges the youngsters come up against and have to master in their everyday lives. We can teach children from early on via developing our own breath awareness and competence in the areas of health and wellbeing.

At the End and at the Start

Breathing correctly cannot be considered insignificant for our health and inner balance. We breathe in and out about 25 000 times per day, all through our live from birth to death. In this book, you have encountered important new insights, which have helped us to understand more about our breathing and to direct it in an orientation, which best suits our organism.

The secret of correct breathing has been revealed, at least a little bit. We now know how we can influence our nervous system by our breathing and thus increase our inner stability and foundation for ongoing well-being.

The message of this book is this: You can act beneficially for your health and inner balance at any moment: Breathe in a coherent rhythm. This also helps you to be more beneficial to others, for in a state of coherence you can be more open, friendly and amiable. When something upsets you, you now know how to quickly come back to yourself and your inner safety and calmness: Breathe regularly, relaxed and slowly, in your own coherent rhythm.

When you like other breathing exercises, enjoy them and remember Coherent Breathing as soon as you return to normal breathing. With sufficient practice in Coherent Breathing, it will gradually become your normal way of breathing, and this means that inner coherence will steadily become your normal condition.

So, I want to encourage you to adopt Coherent Breathing. You can practice the method in its simple, basic form as presented in this book or move on to researching and measuring your own individual resonance frequency. The central point of this method is consistent practice, and for this I wish you a lot of perseverance and creativity to find as many opportunities to practice as possible in your life.

If you have questions to the method or any feedback to this book, you can contact me at info@wilfried-ehrmann.com. You find information for my therapeutic work and seminars at www.wilfried-ehrmann.com.

Glossary

Acetylcholine: messenger substance for attention and learning, transmitted by the parasympathicus to the sinus node to slow down the heartbeat.

Adrenalin: hormone for initiating the stress reaction. With the perception of a stress related stimulus, the hypothalamus activates the sympathicus, and then the adrenal medulla releases adrenaline.

Aerobic Dissimilation (=inner breathing): decomposition of endogenous organic compounds for generating energy by means of oxygen on the cellular level.

Alkalosis: blood is alkaline with a pH-value above 7.44.

Autonomic (Vegetative) Nervous System (ANS): regulates the inner processes in the organism, which cannot be influenced by will. Subdivisions: sympathicus, parasympathicus and enteric nervous system.

Acidosis: blood is acidic with a pH-value below 7.36.

Baroreceptor: mechanical measure points of blood pressure at the arterial vascular walls.

> **Baroreceptor reflex**: stabilizing the arterial blood pressure by a feedback loop. It reduces the heart frequency with increased blood pressure and vice versa.

Biofeedback: Method for visualizing physical functions with the aim of self-regulation by operant conditioning.

Bohr-Effect: stronger attachment of oxygen to hemoglobin when the blood becomes too alkaline (by exhaling CO_2), which hampers the release of oxygen to the body cells.

Brain Stem: oldest part of the brain, regulates basic metabolic processes like breathing and blood circulation.

Cerebrospinal Fluid (CSF, liquor cerebrospinalis): serves as padding of brain and spinal cord and cleanses the brain from debris mainly during sleep.

Coherence: physics: tendency of waves to find a shared vibration.

> **Breath - Heart Coherence**: attunement of breathing and heart frequency.

> **Heart Coherence**: regular changes of → R-R-intervals.

Sense of Coherence: most important resource for → Salutogenesis: understanding reality, mastering challenges and fostering positive meaning.

Control pause: method for self-checking the pH-value in the blood by measuring the maximal length of holding the breath.

Cortisol: stress hormone, inhibits the immune system, produced in the adrenal cortex.

Distress: unhealthy or detrimental stress; chronic stress

DHEA: Dehydroepiandrosterone, steroid hormone, produced in the adrenal cortex, precursor of sexual hormones.

Dopamine: messenger substance for stimulation, attention and learning aptitude, also connected to the gratification centers in the brain.

EMDR (=Eye Movement Desensitization and Reprocessing): method of trauma therapy, in which the client follows the movements of the therapist's hand.

Eustress: stress experience, which is beneficial for our health, or stress in a controlled environment or the adaptability of the organism to varying conditions.

Epigenetics: branch of science occupied with the factors for switching genes on and off, and with changes in the genes, which are not brought about by mutation and yet are transferred from generation to generation.

Expansive Feelings: Feelings like joy, pleasure, interest, curiosity.

First-Person-Perspective: perception of reality by senses turned inwardly e.g. by introspection or self-reflection.

Gamma-Amino-Butter-Acid (GABA): Messenger substance, inter alia in charge of over-reactions of the nervous system.

Heart rate variability: variation in the time interval between heartbeats. Indicator for health and regenerative ability.

Homoeostasis: self-regulation, generation of inner balance.

Hormesis: beneficial reaction to small doses of detrimental influences, e.g. toxins or stress; in the context of endurance sports and physical exercises as beneficial effects of moderate stress.

Hypoxia: undersupply of tissue with oxygen.

Mitochondrion: cellular organelle for generating energy.

Nitrogen Monoxide (NO): gas produced inter alia in the sinuses, has delating effects in vessels and inhibits inflammation.

Noradrenaline: messenger substance and hormone to trigger the stress reaction, released by the adrenal medulla just as adrenalin. It is also produced in the brain.

Oxytocin: messenger substance and hormone, inter alia responsible for lowering blood pressure and cortisol level, has calming and stress reductive effects, also known as "attachment hormone".

Para-Power: performance of the parasympathetic nervous system, measurable by heart rate variability.

Parasympathicus: calming and regenerating part of the autonomic nervous system.

Polyvagal Theory: model of the vegetative nervous system with two functionally and anatomically different parts of the vagus nerve. The evolutionary younger part regulates the social systems in mammals and humans.

Procedural Memory=implicit memory: memory for storing behavioral patterns, which run automatically; also unconscious contents from preverbal developmental phases are attributed to this storage.

Protective Feelings: feelings like fear, anger, pain and disgust, predominantly regulated by the sympathicus.

Resilience: ability to master challenges and activate resources so that crisis can become chances for development.

Resonance Frequency: breathing frequency providing optimal results of heart rate variability, differs from person to person.

Respiratory Arterial Pressure (RAP): Connection between breathing, autonomic nervous system and arterial blood pressure.

Respiratory Generator: a center in the brain stem hypothesized by cardiologists for regulating breathing in accordance with the activities of the heart.

Respiratory Sinusarrhythmia: increase of heart frequency with inhalation, decrease with exhalation. This phenomenon is stronger with slow breathing.

rpm=respiration per minute

R-R-Interval: temporal difference between two R-spikes on the ECG.

Salutogenesis: approach focusing on the aspects which promote health instead of those which make sick.

Serotonin: messenger substance, regulates the tension in the blood vessels and has a positive impact on the emotional mood.

Sinu-atrial Node: renders impulses for the heartbeat, modulated by parasympathicus.

Sympathicus: activating part of the autonomic nervous system.

System Social Engagement (SSE): regulates social behavior based on the activities of the new vagus → polyvagal theory.

Third-Person-Perspective: Reality as perceived by the outward directed senses, also with the help of instruments for measurement.

Thorax Pump: movement of breathing with the diaphragm and thorax as third power for moving the blood flow besides heart and arteria.

Total-Power: Total performance of the frequency bands in HRV-measurement, gives information about the strength of sympathicus and parasympathicus.

Vagus: tenth brain nerve originating from the brain stem, innerving the parasympathicus. The dorsal (retral) part forms the old vagal system, the ventral (front) part forms the new vagal system → polyvagal theory.

> **Vagale Brake**: restrictive influence of the ventral vagus on the sympathicus for calming heartbeat and stress reaction.

Valsalva-Wave: rise and fall of pressure in the circulatory system connected with the increase and decrease of heart frequency with the breathing movement as central impulse generator.

Vasopressin: hormone with vasoconstrictive effects, regulates blood pressure and takes part in coupling.

Bibliography

Antonovsky, Aaron: Health, Stress and Coping. San Francisco: Jossey-Bass Publishers 1979

Bauer, Joachim: Warum ich fühle, was du fühlst. Intuitive Kommunikation und das Geheimnis der Spiegelneurone. Hamburg: Hoffmann und Campe 2005

Blackett, Glyn: Mind-Body Intelligence. How to Manage Your Mind Using Biofeedback & Mindfulness. Colin Glyn Blackett 2014

Boll-Klatt, Annegret & Kohrs, Mathias: Praxis der psychodynamischen Psychotherapie: Grundlagen - Modelle – Konzepte. Stuttgart: Schattauer 2013

Brown, Richard P. & Gerbarg, Patricia L.: Sudarshan Kriya Yogic Breathing in the Treatment of Stress, Anxiety, and Depression .PartII–clinical applications and guidelines. J. Altern. Complement. Med. 11, 711–717, 2005

Brown, Richard P. & Gerbarg, Patricia L.: The Healing Power of the Breath. Boston: Shambala 2012

Chamberlain David: Windows to the Womb: Revealing the Conscious Baby from Conception to Birth. Berkeley: North Atlantic Books 2013

Childre, Doc, Martin, Howard & Beech, Donna: The HeartMath Solution: The Institute of HeartMath's Revolutionary Program for Engaging the Power of the Heart's Intelligence. HarperOne, New York 2000

Collings, Peter J.: Liquid Crystals. Nature's Delicate Phase of Matter. Princeton: University Press 2001

Ehrmann, Wilfried: Handbuch der Atemtherapie. Ahlstedt: Param 2004

Ehrmann, Wilfried: Consciousness in Evolution. Bielefeld: Tao 2014

Elliott, Stephen & Edmonson, Dee: Coherent Breathing. The Definitive Method. Theory & Practice. Allen Texas: Coherence Press 2008

Elliott, Stephen: Personal Resonance Protocol With Coherence Valsalva Wave Pro. An Instruction Manual. Allen Texas: Coherence Press 2016a

Elliott, Stephen: Circulatory Physiology 101: What You Don't Know Can Hurt You. Swan & Stone, Volume 1, Issue 7, 2016b

Faller, Norbert: Atem und Bewegung. Theorie und 111 Übungen. Wien: Springer Verlag 2009

Grimm, Melanie: Heartness®. Das holistische Herzbewusstsein entdecken. Berlin: ProBusiness 2015

Grof Stanislav: The Adventure of Self-Discovery: Dimensions of Consciousness and New Perspectives In Psychotherapy. State Univ of New York Press 1988

Harrer, Michael E. & Weiss, Halko: Wirkfaktoren der Achtsamkeit – wie sie die Psychotherapie verändern und bereichern. Stuttgart: Schattauer 2016

Hidas, György & Raffai, Jenö: Nabelschnur der Seele: Psychoanalytische orientierte Förderung der vorgeburtlichen Bindung zwischen Mutter und Baby (psychosozial) 2006

Hof, Wim & Rosales, Justin: Becoming the Iceman. Minneapolis: Mill City Press 2011

Hüther, Gerald & Sachsse, Ulrich (2007): Neurobiologisch fundierte Psycho-therapie. In: Dammann Gerald, Janssen Paul L. (ed.) Psychotherapie der Border-line-Störungen. Thieme Stuttgart and New York, 129-142

Iyengar B.K.S.: Light on Pranayama. The Yogic Art of Breathing. New York: Crossroad 1994

Janov, Arthur: Life Before Birth: The Hidden Script that Rules our Lives. Portland: NTI Upstream 2011

Janus, Ludwig: Der Seelenraum des Ungeborenen - Pränatale Psychologie und Therapie. Ostfildern: Patmos 2011

Judith Kravitz: Breathe Deep, Laugh Loudly. The Joy of Transformational Breathing. Free Breath Press 2002

Lehrer, Paul M. & Gevirtz, Richard: Heart Rate Variability Biofeedback: How and Why does it Work? Frontiers in Psychology, July 2014, Volume 5, Article 756

Lorenz, Rüdiger: Salutogenese: Grundwissen für Psychologen, Mediziner, Gesundheits- und Pflegewissenschaftler. München and Basel: Verlag Reinhardt 2005

Lucas, Marsha: Rewire Your Brain for Love: Creating Vibrant Relationships Using the Science of Mindfulness. Carlsbad: Hay House 2012

McKeown, Patrick: Close Your Mouth. Buteyko Clinic Self Help Manual. Asthma Care: Galway 2011

McKeown, Patrick: The Oxygen Advantage: The Simple, Scientifically Proven Breathing Techniques for a Healthier, Slimmer, Faster, and Fitter You. William Morrow: New York 2015

Middendorf, Ilse: The Perceptible Breath: A Breathing Science. Paderborn: Junfermann 1990

Minett Gunnel: Breath & Spirit: Rebirthing as a Healing Technique. London: Harpercollins 1994

Müller-Schwefe, Rudolf: EMDR und Körper-Psychotherapie: Ein neuer Zugang zum salutogenen Prozess. In: Psychoanalyse & Körper Nr. 10, 6.Jg., Heft 1. Berlin: Psychosozial Verlag 2007

Narayanananda Swami: The Secrets of Prana, Pranayama and Yoga-Asanas. Gylling: Narayana Press 1979

Ogden, Pat, Minton, Kekuni & Pain, Clare: Trauma and the Body. A Sensorimotor Approach to Psychotherapy. New York/London: Norton 2006

Olsson, Anders: The Power of Your Breath. Tallinna, Estonia 2014

Platteel-Deur, Tilke: The Art of Integrative Therapy: Healing the Past on a Soul Level. BookRix 2014

Porges, Stephen W.: The Polyvagal Theory: Neurophysiologial Foundations of Emotions, Attachment, Communication, and Self-regulation. New York: W. W. Norton & Company 2011; cit. from the German edition: Die Polyvagal-Theorie. Neurophysiologische Grundlagen der Therapie. Paderborn: Junfermann 2010

Rank, Otto: The Trauma of Birth (orig. 1924). Eastford: Martino Fine Books 2010

Das Trauma der Geburt: und seine Bedeutung für die Psychoanalyse (1924). Berlin: Psychosozial-Verlag 2007

Renggli, Franz: Das goldene Tor zum Leben: Wie unser Trauma aus Geburt und Schwangerschaft ausheilen kann. München: Arkana 2013

Roth, Gerhard & Strüber, Nicole: Wie das Gehirn die Seele macht. Stuttgart: Klett-Cotta 2014

Ruppert, Franz: Frühes Trauma. Schwangerschaft, Geburt und erste Lebensjahre. Stuttgart: Klett-Cotta 2014

Sabatini, Sandra: Breath: The Essence of Yoga. London: Pinter & Martin 2007

Servan-Schreiber, David: The Instinct to Heal: Curing Depression, Anxiety, and Stress Without Drugs and Without Talk Therapy. Emmaus: Rodale Books, 2004

Schmidt, Johannes B.: Der Körper kennt den Weg. Trauma-Heilung und persönliche Transformation. München: Kösel 2008

Siegel, Daniel J.: The Healing Power of Emotion: Affective Neuroscience, Development & Clinical Practice (New York: WW Norton & Company, 2009)

Van der Kolk, Bessel: Verkörperter Schrecken. Traumaspuren in Gehirn, Geist und Körper und wie man sie heilen kann. Lichtenau/Westfalen: Probst 2015

Watkins, Alan: Coherence. The Secret Science of Brilliant Leadership. London: Kogan Page 2014

Weineck, Jürgen: Sportbiologie. Balingen: Spitta Verlag 2004

Wittling, Werner & Wittling, Ralf Arne: Heart rate variability: Frühwarnsystem, Stress- und Fitnessindikator. Heiligenstadt: Eichsfeldverlag 2012

Wydler, Hans, Kolip, Petra & Abel, Thomas (ed.): Salutogenese und Kohärenzgefühl. Grundlagen, Empirie und Praxis eines gesundheitswissenschaftlichen Konzepts. Weinheim München: Juventa 2010

List of Figures

References

1 Negrao BL1, Bipath P, van der Westhuizen D, Viljoen M: Autonomic correlates at rest and during evoked attention in children with attention-deficit/ hyperactivity disorder and effects of methylphenidate. Neuropsychobiology. 2011;63(2):82-91. doi: 10.1159/000317548. Epub 2010 Dec 18. http://www.ncbi.nlm.nih.gov/pubmed/21178382, 2.2.2016

2 http://upliftconnect.com/control-inflammation/12.4.2016

3 http://clearingtrauma.homestead.com, 4.2.2016

4 Mae-Wan Ho in: http://www.i-sis.org.uk/brainde.php, 31.1.2016 (Übersetzung: Wilfried Ehrmann)

5 https://www.siam.org/pdf/news/353.pdf

6 E. Baulieu, G. Thomas et al.: Dehydroepiandrosterone (DHEA) DHEA sulfate, and aging:contribution of the DHEAge Study to a soziobiomedical issue. In: Proc Natal Acad Sci USA, Bd 97 (8), 2000, S. 4279-4284

7 WA Tiller, R McCraty, M. Atkinson Cardiac coherence: a new, noninvasive measure of autonomic nervous system order. In: Altern Ther Health Med., 1996 Jan, 2(1), S. 52–65, PMID 8795873. Department of Materials Science and Engineering, Stanford University, California, USA, 8.2.2016

8 http://www.dr-guenter.de/images/pp/hrv_messung.pdf, 18.12.2015

9 www.pulse.or.at/downloads/hrv-im-sportcoaching.pdf, 6.12.2015

10 Quelle: http://www.hrv24.de/HRV-Lexikon.htm, 6.12.2015

11 http://www.ncbi.nlm.nih.gov/pubmed/12624607, 18.11.2015

12 stroke.ahajournals.org/content/42/11/3196.full.pdf, 16.11.2015

13 http://www.ncbi.nlm.nih.gov/pmc/articles/PMC3446945, 21.9.2015

14 Hier findet sich eine recht harsche, aber stichhaltige Kritik von Scott Alexander an der Methode und dem Marketing von HeartMath: http://slatestarcodex.com/2014/07/17/heartmath-considered-incoherent, 4.6.2015

15 https://www.ncbi.nlm.nih.gov/pubmed/18951492

16 http://erj.ersjournals.com/content/22/2/323, 27.1.2016

17 http://www.york-biofeedback.co.uk/blog/index.php/388/is-mindfulness-the-best-way-to-boost-heart-rate-variability, 25.1.2016

18 www.coherence.com/The_Six_Bridges_Revisited.pdf, 18.1.2017

19 http://www.holographic-breathing.com, 16.5.2016

20 http://www.kirsten-heinrich.de/download/HRV_Diagnostik_Comed_ 0608.pdf, 15.4.2016

21 http://www.icemanwimhof.com/science, 1.2.2016

22 http://www.ncbi.nlm.nih.gov/pubmed/11253418, 30.3.2016

23 http://maps.cancer.gov/overview/DCCPSGrants/abstract.jsp?applId=8641669&term=CA163640, 29.11.2015, 4.2.2016

24 http://thoughtbrick.com/wim-hof-method/wim-hof-method-power-breath-exercise-explained/, 18.1.17

25 Mück-Weymann, M., et al.: Depression modulates autonomic cardiac control: a physiological pathway linking depression and mortality? German J. Psychiatry 2002 (5) 67-69; Mück-Weymann, M., et al.: Do depression symptoms affect autonomic control of the heart? Clinical Autonomic Research 2000 (10) 244-245

26 http://www.nature.com/tp/journal/v6/n2/full/tp2015225a.html, 22.2.2016

27 D. Löllgen, M. Mück-Weymann, R. Beise: Herzratenvariabilitäts-Biofeedback in der betrieblichen Gesundheitsförderung – Eine Pilotstudie. (PDF) Forum Stressmedizin 2009, 22.2.2016

28 http://www.nature.com/tp/journal/v6/n2/full/tp2015225a.html, 23.2.2016

29 http://www.netdoktor.at/krankheit/antidepressiva-anstieg-oesterreich-6866981, 24.2.2016

The Author:
Wilfried Ehrmann, PhD

Psychotherapist working with breathing, trauma healing and prenatal therapy, practicing in Vienna.

International seminar leader and trainer for therapeutic breathwork, mindfulness trainer and lecturer.
Numerous publications and blog articles about breath therapy, philosophy, psychotherapy, spirituality and integral practice.

Website: **www.wilfried-ehrmann.com**

English blogsite: **https://wilfried-ehrmann-e.blogspot.com**

To the Forum for this book: **http://tao.de/users/wilfried-ehrmann**

Further book in English:
Consciousness in Evolution. Tao 2014

Books in German:
Handbuch der Atemtherapie 2004

Vom Mut zu wachsen 2011

Vierzig Tore der Weisheit 2015